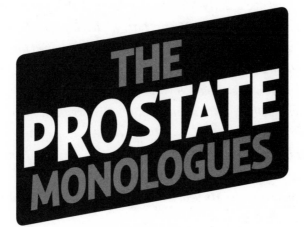

Also by Jack McCallum

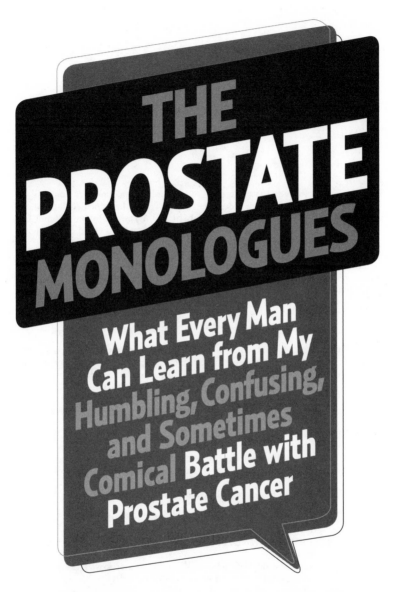

THE PROSTATE MONOLOGUES

What Every Man Can Learn from My Humbling, Confusing, and Sometimes Comical Battle with Prostate Cancer

JACK McCALLUM

RODALE.

Rodale books may be purchased for business or promotional use or for special sales.
For information, please write to:
Special Markets Department, Rodale Inc., 733 Third Avenue, New York, NY 10017.

Printed in the United States of America
Rodale Inc. makes every effort to use acid-free ♾, recycled paper ♺.

Book design by George Karabotsos

Excerpt from AMERICAN PASTORAL by Philip Roth.
Copyright © 1997 by Philip Roth. Used by permission of
Houghton Mifflin Harcourt Publishing Company. All rights reserved.

Library of Congress Cataloging-in-Publication Data is on file with the publisher.
ISBN-13: 978-1-60961-055-5   hardcover

Distributed to the trade by Macmillan

2   4   6   8   10   9   7   5   3   1   hardcover

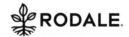

We inspire and enable people to improve their lives and the world around them.
rodalebooks.com

To GEORGE B. YASSO
*Who died too soon of prostate cancer
but who got a lot done while he was here*

*"If treatment for cure is necessary, is it possible?
If possible, is it necessary?"*

—WILLET WHITMORE, MD,

famed urologist and prostate cancer victim,
on the problematic nature of treating prostate cancer

Contents

CONTENTS

CONTENTS

Prologue

While we waited for dessert, the Swede let pass that he was indulging himself in a fattening zabaglione on top of the ziti only because, after having had his prostate removed a couple of months back, he was still some ten pounds underweight.

"The operation went okay?"

"Just fine," he replied.

"A couple friends of mine," I said, "didn't emerge from that surgery as they'd hoped to. That operation can be a real catastrophe for a man, even if they get the cancer out."

"Yes, that happens, I know."

"One wound up impotent," I said. "The other's impotent and incontinent. Fellows my age. It's been rough for them. Desolating. It can leave you in diapers."

—PHILIP ROTH, *American Pastoral*

GIVEN THE RESERVOIR OF DISPIRITING SUBJECTS explored by Philip Roth over his long career, it is not surprising that his fictional alter ego, Nathan Zuckerman, came upon prostate cancer in this 1997 novel that won the Pulitzer Prize for Fiction. You want to get any man depressed, just bring up the sometimes intertwined complications of uncontrollable urinary function and insufficient erections and watch him grab his favorite NFL sponge toy and retreat to his man cave.

Let me make it clear that I have had the same operation as Roth's protagonist, Seymour "Swede" Levov, and, like the Swede, "I got off easy."

Kind of easy, anyway. I'm still trying to figure that out, as you'll see in the succeeding chapters. With this disease, see, you rarely get off easy. Even if you're not peeing like a one-year-old or having trouble "in the bedroom" as the commercials describe it, your eardrums are being assaulted by a Greek chorus of second-guessers.

"You shouldn't have got it done! You shouldn't have got it done!" Prostate cancer intervention has become in some quarters a kind of cosmetic surgery, the glandular counterpart to the nose job. To an increasing number of people both within and without the medical profession, prostate is the friendly cancer, so unlike pancreatic, brain, breast, and lung, and much more benevolent than its brothers, testicular and bladder. You can live a long time with prostate cancer. Just about every man in the universe will get it and he probably won't die of it. *"Why the hell did you make yourself impotent when you didn't have to?"*

Ah, but choose to live with prostate cancer instead of having it excised or irradiated and you hear a different chorus: "It's still cancer. Any cancer can kill you. Advanced prostate cancer is as bad as any other kind of cancer. *Why the hell are you risking death by doing nothing!"*

The two sides are locked in a debate that conjures up *Rashomon*, the celebrated Akira Kurosawa movie in which different characters relate incompatible versions of the same story. Mounds of data speak to the key questions of the prostate debate: How effective is PSA testing? At what age should men start to get tested? Does PSA testing prevent deaths? What is the best way to treat prostate cancer?—but myriad ways of interpreting them. It is a medical Rorschach: One expert sees this, another sees that, a third sees something else. And when experts can't agree, it leaves the nonexpert in a quandary, as we are when we try to sift through conflicting investment advice.

At the very least, though, those of us in the Prostate Cancer Club can take pride that we clearly have the "It" malignancy, the male version of breast cancer, if you will. That is not a comment on the comparative severity of the diseases; it is merely to note that prostate—while lacking a Susan G. Komen–like standard-bearer, the full-blown, pink-gloved, fund-raising partnership of the National Football League and a thousand weekend benefit runs—is the cancer that these days is commanding much of the attention and almost all of the controversy.

President Barack Obama declared September 2012 the first Prostate Cancer Awareness Month in the United States. Two months later, there's another way to recognize prostate cancer—"Movember." It's a movement that began a decade ago in Australia in which men grow mustaches (a "mo" is Aussie shorthand for one) for men's health awareness, and it has now raised millions of dollars and has the official sanction of the Prostate Cancer Foundation. That organization was founded by the disease's deep-pocketed champion, Michael Milken, the junk bond villain turned medical philanthropist who is himself a prostate cancer survivor.

The Lehigh Valley Iron Pigs, a minor league baseball team in my area, has been active in prostate cancer awareness, combining ads from Urology Specialists of the Lehigh Valley with a foam finger giveaway, a not-so-subtle reminder that a doctor's finger goes along with the digital rectal exam. The Iron Pigs have also added a "Urinal Gaming System" in all of their bathrooms at Coca-Cola Park. Men aim their stream to compete in various games, the scores of which can then be entered and—get this—posted on the scoreboard for all to see. The system was added in conjunction with the Lehigh Valley Health Network with the express purpose of raising prostate awareness. Whether that will happen is a matter of conjecture, but there is little doubt that it has garnered the Pigs a huge amount of national publicity and a torrent of puns. *Streaming media. Bladder up. Whiz Kids.* You get the point.

Even at a Jethro Tull concert these days you're liable to get a prostate reminder (blessedly brief) orchestrated by flautist Ian Anderson, who has fronted the group since I was listening to them nearly five decades ago in college. A plant in the audience gets up in midsong, presumably to urinate, and Anderson calls attention to him. This leads to a skit, visible by shadowy pantomime behind a curtain, in which a man gets a digital rectal exam as Anderson talks about the importance of getting tested and images of rock performers Frank Zappa and Johnny Ramone flash on a video screen. Both died of the disease.

Still, there are other worlds for the prostate people to explore. They have not, for example, been as creative as advocates for another type of cancer who in March of 2013 managed to put up a 20-foot-long walk-through colon in New York City's Times Square for National Colorectal Cancer Awareness Month. "Kids, after we see the Statue of Liberty and the Empire State Building, your father wants to visit the Giant Colon."

IN A WAY, I'll be trying to do in this book what Ian Anderson tries to do in his concerts—tell you a few things without being preachy (and without a digital rectal reenactment). I will tell you about prostate cancer in general, not because I went to med school, which I did not, but because of firsthand experience, research, and interviews with urologists, cancer experts, and other members of the Prostate Cancer Club. I will tell you a number of doctors' opinions on treating prostate cancer, and, as you'll discover, they do not speak with a united voice.

I will tell you about my cancer. I will tell you about my operation and an operation just like mine that I witnessed. I will tell you about my postsurgical complications.

I will tell you a lot about other people's cancers and their complications. I will tell you about the people who say I did the right thing and the people who say I did the wrong thing, and why each says what they say. I will tell you about the Gleason score and percentage of core involvement, as well as some facts about PSA (prostate-specific

antigen), ED (erectile dysfunction), BPH (benign prostatic hyperplasia, a fancy term for an enlarged prostate), DRE (digital rectal
exam), and whatever other combinations of the prostate alphabet
come into play.

Here's what I will not do: If you've already had surgery or radiation, I will not tell you that you did the wrong thing. (Though others I
interviewed might do that.) If you've decided to do nothing and instead
monitor your prostate cancer, I will not tell you that you're doing the
wrong thing. If you're about to have intervention, surgery, radiation,
or anything else, I will not tell you that you're making a big mistake.

This is a book about information and options, probabilities and
statistics, ideas and outcomes—not lectures and regrets. You don't
have to look far, after all, to get plenty of those.

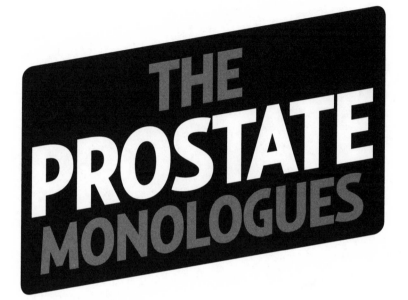

CHAPTER 1

... In which the author hears about an orgasm, lays out the prostate stats, witnesses a prostatectomy, and against all odds does not lose his lunch

THE CALL CAME IN AT ABOUT 10:00 P.M. It was Asha Jagtiani, a woman I had met only once, delivering the following information:

"Jack," she said, "Leonard wanted me to tell you that he just had an orgasm. He is very, very happy."

"That's fantastic," I said. "Tell me about it."

"We were fooling around," said Asha, "and it just happened. We didn't really expect much but then, all of a sudden, he said he orgasmed."

"It was dry, right?" I asked.

"Oh, yes," said Asha. "Nothing came out. But he said it felt just like an orgasm and we wanted you to know. This has made him feel even better about the operation, the fact that he can still have sexual relations."

"I understand completely," I said. "Tell Leonard congratulations."

I am not a close pal of Leonard Collier's, I am not a sex counselor, and I am not Dr. Phil. When I received this climactic news, I had never met Leonard Collier personally, though I had seen him knocked out cold and stripped down naked in a refrigerated operating room. Our connection is this: I had watched Leonard go through the same surgical procedure (robotic prostatectomy) performed by the same surgeon (David Lee, MD) at the same hospital (Penn Presbyterian Medical Center in Philadelphia) that I had gone through. Those who have endured prostatectomy surgery often compare notes.

This was a happy one.

THREE WEEKS BEFORE ASHA'S ORGASM NEWS, I am sitting in the office of said Dr. Lee, the chief of urology at Penn Presbyterian Medical Center, early on a Wednesday morning. In about an hour he will be sitting behind the console of a $1.9 million robotic device, a multi-tentacled thing that resembles a droid from *Star Wars*, directing its "fingers" as it cuts into the abdomen of Collier, a 64-year-old retired educator from West Chester, Pennsylvania.

But at this moment, Dr. Lee is thinking about golf.

"Putting," he says, "is much harder than what I'm about to do. Putting is mysterious."

Putting is mysterious, I agree. But so is surgery. And so is the concept of digging into someone's abdominal cavity and pulling out a gland through a small hole just above the navel—especially because it's done without the surgeon actually touching the man or even standing over him.

I'm a little nervous. I'm not a huge fan of blood and gore, my own or anyone else's. I never wanted to be a doctor, never even played doctor. The robotic prostatectomy procedure is available for viewing on the Penn Web site and, like everything else in the world, on YouTube, but I had chosen not to watch one before my own surgery. Still, research is research, so here I am, scrubbing up and trying to figure out how to carry notebook, pen, and tape recorder into an operating room without dropping them into Leonard Collier's abdominal cavity.

I should emphasize that Leonard, just now going blithely and utterly to sleep in the prep room, does not object to my being there; a week earlier he had given me permission to watch his innards being opened up. To the extent that one can be gung ho about surgery, that state of mind would describe Leonard, who, as an African American, is aware of the greater risk he faces of dying of prostate cancer. Nor would Leonard object to the pre-procedure, off-topic talk about golf: He had selected Dr. Lee not only because of the surgeon's experience (3,300 robotic prostatectomies), but also because Lee is a fellow golfing traveler.

It is difficult to get precise numbers, but Leonard Collier's prostate and mine were two of somewhere between 55,000 and 75,000 that were removed in 2012 across these United States. About 25 percent of men with cancerous prostates chose to intervene with various forms of radiation. A much smaller number chose to monitor their cancer without surgical or radiological intervention in what is known as "active surveillance." A 2010 article in the *Journal of Clinical Oncology* reported that 7 percent of the men in a particular study chose that route, so that would put the 2012 active-surveillance number at roughly between 3,850 and 5,250.

The reason that there is so much prostate cancer activity is that there is so much prostate cancer. The National Cancer Institute (NCI) predicted that about 241,740 new cases of prostate cancer would be diagnosed in 2012 (final numbers were not yet available at the time of this writing), making it the second most common cancer in men behind skin cancer. The NCI estimated that prostate cancer would kill 28,170 men in the same year, making it the second-leading cause of death in men behind lung cancer, which would likely kill 87,750 men (and 72,590 women). Overall, prostate cancer is responsible for 3 percent of all male deaths.

But parse those numbers carefully. First, don't conflate 28,170 with 241,740; most of the deaths are from cancers that were diagnosed much earlier than 2011. Prostate cancer is among the slowest growing of all cancers, with an estimated 80 percent of the cases nonaggressive and slow growing (meaning a nettlesome 20 percent—a not insignificant number—are aggressive).

Second, relatively few of the men diagnosed die of the disease. By comparison, the NCI estimated that in 2012 there would be 43,920 new cases of pancreatic cancer and 37,390 deaths. Not all of the newly diagnosed died within one year, but the best estimate from the American Cancer Society is that the five-year survival rate for pancreatic is only 4 percent. By contrast, the 15-year survival rate for prostate cancer is above 90 percent. Perhaps "I have prostate cancer" sometimes sounds so horrific because it's heard as "I have pancreatic cancer." Misidentification through alliteration.

Look at it this way: About 1 in 6 men will be diagnosed with prostate cancer at some time in his life, but only 1 in 36 will die of the disease. Of course, if your loved one is that "1," you don't think of it as an "only" number.

Prostate cancer is considered an old man's disease, and there is much truth to that. The probability of being diagnosed with prostate cancer is 1 in 8,499 for men younger than 40; 1 in 38 for men ages 40 through 59; 1 in 15 for men ages 60 through 69; and 1 in 8 for men ages 70 and older. About 70 percent of men who die from prostate cancer are older than 75.

But what does that mean exactly? A 75-year-old man was considered absolutely ancient by our forefathers. If you want to live to, say, 95—and at present I have no reason to think I don't—75 isn't all that old. According to the US Census Bureau, the average white male lives almost 8 years longer (75.9 years compared to 68) now than he did in 1970, and the average black male lives almost 11 years longer (70.9 years instead of 60).

None of those statistics recommend for or against treatment. They are merely more things to toss into the cluttered prostate cancer options bag.

As I wrote in the Prologue, prostate cancer has an increasingly high public profile. Lung cancer is far more deadly, but gets far less attention. "It's the blame thing," says Peter Bach, MD, a lung cancer specialist and attending physician at Memorial Sloan-Kettering Cancer Center in New York City. "Lung cancer affects people who are poor, first of all, because it lines up with smoking. And there aren't a lot of survivors. There are a lot of survivors of prostate cancer."

Actually, prostate cancer, according to some researchers, is much more closely linked with the environment and lifestyle than people think. Asian men hardly ever die of prostate cancer, for example, though they develop it in greater numbers when they emigrate to Western countries, possibly as a result of changes in diet and an uptick in stress.

Because a relatively small percentage of diagnosed men die of prostate cancer, there has long been a movement among those with low-risk cases not to treat it, and to instead adopt a "watch and wait" philosophy. In the February 2004 issue of *The Lancet Oncology*, a British medical journal, Chris Parker, MD, described prostate cancer as "the only human cancer that is curable but which commonly does not need to be cured." Much debate is taking place—and will be covered in this book—about what qualifies as "commonly."

The numbers are again hazy, but there will probably be more who choose not to get treated in 2013 than there were in 2012, and there likely will be more in 2014 than there were in 2013. If "active surveillance" can't be characterized as a full-scale march, it certainly seems to be a mobilization. And as the calendar carries me further away from February 20, 2012, the date of my robotic prostatectomy, I will continue to wonder if I should have joined that active-surveillance movement. I don't agonize about it, but I wonder.

I DON'T RECALL anything about my robotic procedure, of course, having drifted peacefully into anesthetic purgatory just as Dr. Lee and I were talking about getting together to play golf. I awakened a few hours later, having lost from my body weight 39 grams—about 1.4 ounces—the weight of my average-sized cancerous prostate.

So I am going to witness Leonard's surgery to see what was done to me.

Kelly Monahan, Dr. Lee's PA (physician assistant), escorts me into Operating Room 9, which is much larger than a meat locker though not a helluva lot warmer. Dead-to-the-world Leonard Collier is lying spread-eagle on a small table and three nurses and a resident are prepping him for surgery, lining the table with protective gauze, checking instrument calibrations, peppering the cool, sterile air with medical gobbledygook.

This is the moment—before surgery—that sticks with me most viscerally. Leonard Collier looks so . . . so . . . vulnerable, all the more so when the Torquemadian leg spreader is activated. I can't help imagining what I looked like in a room that cold (let us never forget the *Seinfeld* episode about shrinkage), and in a position that revealing.

"When I was in here, I was all covered up, right?" I ask Kelly.

"Oh, absolutely," she says with a smile. "We didn't see a thing."

Dr. Lee enters the room almost unobtrusively. He is a powerful man around Penn Presbyterian, a rainmaker who performs more than 400 robotic prostatectomies per year, but there is about him none of the stereotypical surgeon's swagger. He is The Man without acting like The Man.

"Can we pause for a timeout?" Dr. Lee says. Everyone gets silent.

"This is Leonard Collier," pronounces Dr. Lee. "He is here for a robot-assisted laparoscopic prostatectomy." (That is the professional nomenclature for the robotic procedure, which goes by "RALP" in the medical journals.)

Other voices chime in with particulars: Date of birth. Allergies. The readiness of the instruments.

"It is 8:27 a.m.," says Dr. Lee. And it's time to begin the anatomical dig toward Leonard Collier's prostate.

The robot is wheeled into place at the feet of the patient. The staff has named it Big Sexy for no apparent reason. They talk affectionately of the robot, almost like it's a human being. Then again, it is doing a lot of the work.

Sterile wrap remains around all of Big Sexy except for its six protruding arms. I have relative freedom to roam around the operating room, but have been cautioned to stay away from both the robot ("Don't even let your hair touch it," Dr. Lee admonishes me) and the instruments ("Jack, you get close to my instruments," says nurse Felicia Wrice in a faux menacing tone, "I'm going to put you to work").

Before Dr. Lee begins the robotic procedure, Leonard's abdomen is basically turned into a pincushion by Kelly and Shailen Sehgal, MD, a resident. They make six small incisions for four robot ports and two laparoscopic instrument ports that will be handled by Kelly. Leonard's abdominal wall must be lifted to allow the insertion of a Veress needle, through which carbon dioxide is pumped into the abdominal cavity, "blowing it up like a balloon," as Dr. Lee describes it, to make more room to operate within.

I ask if this would be harder to do on a younger man with a muscular stomach.

"Absolutely," says Kelly, probably fighting off the temptation to add: "Though it was pretty easy when we did yours."

Kelly and Dr. Sehgal are on either side of Leonard, but when Dr. Lee sits down at the console he is a good seven feet away from the patient. He peers at his screen and begins to work the robot hands. He is seeing a picture of Leonard's abdomen that is magnified 10 times. One of the advantages of robotic surgery is that the surgeon's "physiological tremor" is not a factor in the patient outcome.

The robot's console is equipped with video simulation, but Dr. Lee doesn't find it all that helpful. "Airplane simulators are amazingly close to reality, but it is hard to replicate the body of a living organism," says Dr. Lee. "You need to see blood and tissue deformation." Dr. Lee learned his robotic technique primarily by operating on pigs.

The surgeon eats, plays golf, and stitches with his right hand, but writes and plays tennis with his left. "Being ambidextrous is very beneficial for a surgeon," he says.

As he moves his hands, his right foot also works two pedals. He looks like a cross between a kid playing a video game and an adult playing a church organ. The right pedal is in charge of power, the left is responsible for the motions of the robot. "I only have two hands and there are four robotic instruments," he says, "so I need the pedals."

I ask Dr. Lee, who is in his mid-40s, if he was good at video games. "I have to admit I was," he says. "It seemed to come to me easily. I was right there at the beginning with the Atari system. I remember Space Invaders. And all through medical school it was Tetris."

I am able to watch what Dr. Lee is doing at another console. The picture is 3-D and is so clear and clinical looking that it's not really gross. There is relatively little blood.

There is talk, not constant but steady. "A little more suction, please," Dr. Lee might say. Or "Great, Kelly," after she uses a clip to stanch blood flow. "When you've done as many cases as Dr. Lee and I have done," says Kelly, "there's not a lot of back and forth. Better for us, better for the patient. Less time in the OR, fewer complications."

In the silent spaces I can hear the sonar-sounding *beeps* of the operating room machinery—Leonard's blood pressure (about 112/70) is being monitored by a nurse sitting behind him—and the *snip, snip, snipping* of the robot claws. It's a little eerie. From time to time the lens that is peering into Leonard's abdomen gets dirty and has to be pulled out for a rinse. The nurses spray it with water kept at about 120°F. They don't want it to cool and then fog up when it's returned to the warm body cavity.

The surgeon continues his deliberate advance upon Leonard's prostate, scraping away the fascia that lies on top of the gland, cutting the bladder away from the prostate and dissecting the seminal vesicles. The scene brings to mind the old Raquel Welch movie *Fantastic Voyage* and the similar *Innerspace*. I had been fascinated by the journey through the human body because normally we don't think about what's inside of us.

At one point Kelly says matter-of-factly, "The fat's in the Mayo." What, we're ordering sandwiches now? Actually "the fat" is the layer of fat on the front side of the prostate that Dr. Lee removes, and "the Mayo" is a stand with a tray used to either hold sterilized instruments or collect surgical trash. Dr. Lee had "handed" the fat to Kelly, who removed it from Leonard's abdomen and left it for the scrub nurse. The fat will be sent, along with the prostate and the seminal vesicles—which will be coming out with the gland—to the pathology lab for testing.

The whole scene is one of such calm that I keep forgetting about the danger, the delicacy of the whole thing. Dr. Lee will come close to the obturator nerve at the very top of the inner thigh, and he has to be careful that he doesn't put a hole in Leonard's rectum. Still, he says he considers prostate surgery infinitely less dangerous than, say, kidney surgery, during which he must cut across the renal nerve, which lies atop the aorta.

After about an hour Dr. Lee is ready to cut away the prostate, which he does near the urethra—"the downstream side," as he puts it.

"Big prostate," says Dr. Lee.

"Big prostate," everyone agrees.

That just makes the morning a little more taxing, as it had been when Dr. Lee once had to remove a prostate that weighed 280 grams— about 9.9 ounces—well over a half pound.

"The farther you go down to the tip of the prostate, the tighter and narrower is the space," explains Dr. Lee. "It's like a cone. So when you have guys with really big prostates, there is no room to go from side to side to be able to dissect the tissue away from the prostate." Also, bigger prostates tend to have a more vigorous blood supply, and blood is the enemy of the surgeon.

I feel a surge of relief that my prostate had been so medium-sized and so easily lifted out of the body cavity.

When Dr. Lee finally frees the prostate and the seminal vesicles, they are placed in a plastic bag that had been inserted through one of the ports. The bag is used both because it makes extraction easier and also because it keeps the cancerous prostate from "seeding" cells in other tissues on its way out of the body.

Roughly half of the operation is devoted to getting to the prostate and the other half to stitching. Meanwhile, the bagged prostate remains inside the patient's abdominal cavity, rather like a flounder lying on a dock before being collected and sent to market. The prostate is left there because a slightly larger incision above the navel will have to be made to get it out, and Dr. Lee doesn't want to do that too early lest "we start getting a gas leak."

CHAPTER 1

The stitching continues at a deliberate pace. "What I'm doing now," says Dr. Lee, head buried in the console, "is the Rocco stitch."

"Don't tell me it's named for an Italian surgeon," I said. Not to mention about 173 pizza joints.

"Exactly," he answers. "Now I'm doing a running stitch, going outside-in on the bladder and inside-out on the urethra. Then I run this all the way around to 12 o'clock on the left side and 12 o'clock on the right side." The man loves to stitch, lives to stitch. When he is finished, he will have used 13 stitches to make a watertight connection between Leonard's bladder and urethra. After the prostate is gone, the anatomy in that area is essentially like two pipes with a missing joint: There is a hole in the bladder and a hole in the urethra, and they must be united to restore normal urinary flow.

Finally, Dr. Sehgal wriggles the prostate bag out of Leonard and places it on the Mayo. I stare at it for several seconds.

"I don't care what anybody says," I inform the OR. "Leonard Collier's prostate is a helluva lot bigger than a walnut."

CHAPTER 2

... In which we learn why your prostate is kind of like Liechtenstein

UNTIL A MAN GETS CANCER, his prostate is basically a punch line, a setup prop for a comment about urination, or a comic mispronunciation waiting to happen. *NYPD Blue*, one of TV's great one-hour dramas, got a season's worth of humor out of detective Andy Sipowicz fretting over his "prostrate." This is an understandable mistake, if only because hearing that someone is about to reach inside your rectum and finger-jag your prostate is liable to make a man go prostrate. Throughout the writing of this manuscript, my spell-check software resolutely changed "prostate" to "prostrate" every time, and I sincerely hope that the editors and myself have caught all of them.

Even if you never learn the correct way to say it or spell it, there is one fact about the prostate that will be drummed into your head—its size relative to a salad and sundae staple. For whatever reason, almost every medical professional feels compelled to say, by way of introduction to the gland, some version of the following: "The first thing to know is, your prostate is about the size of a walnut." Back in 1967, J. I. Rodale (the founder of the company that published this book) used the walnut comparison to size up the gland in his book titled, quite logically, *The Prostate.* At least it's easy on the memory—your prostate has much to do with your nuts, so you identify it by association with a nut.

However, there are variations. I read the account of one doctor (presumably from the tropics) who described the prostate as "about the size of a kiwi." Johns Hopkins urologist Patrick Walsh, MD, one of the most important figures in the history of prostate cancer detection and treatment, has been known to compare it to a large strawberry. But in his celebrated book *Dr. Patrick Walsh's Guide to Surviving Prostate Cancer,* Dr. Walsh also uses "walnut," and "walnut" remains the default description. As if to reinforce that, Paulie Gualtieri, one of Tony's associates on *The Sopranos,* required a prostate biopsy in an episode in the show's sixth season. His nickname? Paulie Walnuts.

Humble size notwithstanding, the prostate is strategically located. Its etymology is (of course) Latin, from the Greek *prostates,* which means "one who stands before," a "protector" or "guardian." There is a theory that the prostate evolved to protect the bladder from infection, but in truth, it is as much guarded as guardian. It lies southeast of the bladder and southwest of the rectum. It is wedged between the seminal vesicles and, in a complicated bit of spatial geography, envelops the urethra. So it is most properly described as a walnut being strangled by a garden snake, an ideal symbol, it would seem, for a frightening fundamentalist religion.

"What you have to remember about the prostate," Ballentine Carter, MD, one of Dr. Walsh's preeminent colleagues at Johns Hopkins, told me, "is that it lies in the middle of a lot of valuable real estate." Indeed it does. If there were really such a thing as intelligent design, the prostate would not be so intricately landlocked. Or, alternatively, there would be a little door located at that part of the body, complete with an EJECT button, so the prostate could be easily removed, like an unwatched DVD of *Gigli*.

When a surgeon has to get at the prostate, see, it takes some doing. "All of the anatomy around the prostate is concealed," says Dr. Walsh. And in this hidden location the prostate is rather like doubly land-locked Liechtenstein, a country that nobody talks about or actually visits but is nevertheless somewhat significant because it is bordered by Switzerland and Austria. (Liechtenstein, by the way, is also about the size of a walnut.)

Rather unlike Liechtenstein, however, the prostate actually does something, has a function, doesn't just lie there acting all walnutlike. It is a part of the reproductive system, secreting a slightly acidic fluid through small pores that lie between it and the prostatic urethra. That fluid nourishes and carries sperm as it passes through the urethra on its voyage to wherever the sperm might be headed at the time.

But how much the prostate does is open to debate. Dr. Walsh estimates that it provides only about one-third of the fluid that makes up semen, and, if it stopped producing that entirely, a man might still be able to produce sperm sufficient for fatherhood. Plus, as Leonard Collier and I now know, you don't need the prostate to get or maintain an erection.

Males can achieve orgasm through stimulation of the prostate, though that fact does not come from firsthand observation. An orgasm is the last thing on my mind at that moment when a doctor gives me a digital rectal exam. Technically, I suppose, such a response really isn't an orgasm since—and I haven't completely worked this out yet—orgasm is at least partly a mental act, whereas ejaculation is purely physical. Some men who have trouble ejaculating but want to be fathers choose an operating room procedure in which an electrical probe is passed through their rectum to innervate the prostate, forcing an ejaculation. They are asleep at the time, which is not the normal ejaculatory state, unless you're a 13-year-old experiencing a nocturnal emission.

Testosterone, which is produced in the testicles—better-known prostate neighbors—causes the prostate to grow, which is why stopping testosterone production is often part of the battle against advanced prostate cancer. The simplest way to stop or slow testosterone production is with castration by one of two methods. An early prostate pioneer, Charles B. Huggins, MD, who shared the 1966 Nobel Prize in Physiology or Medicine, is credited with delaying many deaths with hormonal treatments or surgical castration. "The cornerstone treatment for metastatic prostate cancer is still medicinal castration," says Edward Messing, MD, a noted urologist at the University of Rochester Medical Center. But keep in mind that castration is only for these advanced cases, in which the cancer has spread beyond the gland; if you get a diagnosis of localized prostate cancer and a doctor suggests castration, you are in the wrong medical facility and should run immediately for the door marked EXIT.

While you don't need your prostate to urinate, the gland does get involved in the process, not because it's a meddler but because it doesn't have a choice. Again, location, location, location. The urethra, which passes through the prostate on its way from the bladder, is the tube that carries both urine and semen out of the body.

Across the male population, the prostate is much more likely to be involved with urinary issues than with sexual issues. Those of you over 50 are now nodding your heads because you've already had conversations with friends about the epic number of times you get up to pee during the night. As men age, the prostate continues to grow and soon necessitates the use of a different comparator, perhaps even a move from nuts to large-sized fruits. In *The Definitive Guide to Prostate Cancer*, Aaron Katz, MD, writes that a prostate as large as 18 ounces—"the size of two grapefruits"—has been removed from a man. I am still waiting for the first horror film in which a steadily growing prostate escapes the body of a crazed grade school janitor and terrorizes an entire community.

What enlarges the prostate is a condition known as benign prostatic hyperplasia (BPH), though there is nothing benign about a half-dozen trips to the head between midnight and 6:00 a.m. It certainly wasn't convenient if you were one of the Founding Fathers and from time to time had to do your voiding in freezing outhouses—Benjamin Franklin and Thomas Jefferson were said to be BPH sufferers. It turns out that this condition has a name—nocturia, which sounds like the Greek goddess of sleep, and God knows how inappropriate that is.

BPH generally begins in what is known as the prostate's transition zone, the tissue that directly surrounds the urethra. The tissue grows inward, enlarging the gland and constricting the urethra, which restricts urine flow. So you have trouble going, or you go and never quite get it all out and have to get up again to try to finish the job, or you have dribbling after urination (sometimes even double dribbling, a clear violation), or you have pain with urination, a weak urine stream, or blood in your urine.

This marching-off-to-the-head condition is often treated humorously. But it's really not that funny. In January 2013, a California urologist, Ronald Gilbert, MD, was shot and killed in his office by a patient who was reportedly upset over his continued issues with postsurgical incontinence. Also, incontinence is generally treated as a male problem, but it is not. "Men and women have the same urinary issues," says Steven Kaplan, MD, a well-known urologist at NewYork-Presbyterian Hospital and Weill Cornell Medical College. "With men, it pops up in their 50s, and with women, it's generally postmenopausal. Urinating symptoms are going to get everybody sooner or later, and by and large it comes down to what the individual thinks about it. Somebody goes every four hours and maybe it doesn't bother him, but somebody else goes once every six hours and that guy wants a consultation."

As much of an inconvenience as BPH can be, it is not cancer and is far more common. Rodale's book hardly mentions cancer and instead targets the other prostate miseries of enlargement and inflammation. In his seminal medical textbook *Gray's Anatomy*, Henry Gray describes the simple horrors visited by an enlarged prostate. The important thing to remember is that if you have BPH, it doesn't mean you have or will develop cancer, and vice versa. I had cancer but never had BPH, a happenstance I consider a small yet much appreciated miracle. And since I no longer have a prostate, it can't get enlarged, which is one less thing to worry about on my personal road to ruin.

CHAPTER 3

...In which the author for the first time pays real attention to his PSA number

MY FAMILY PHYSICIAN, James Manley, DO, and I had a loose script we followed at my yearly physicals. He would suggest that I get a stress test, and I would say, "Doc, when I go down, I'm going down from the Big C. My heart's fine."

I believed that, too. Cholesterol, heart rate, blood pressure—all those things were always good; I took reasonably good care of what I could take care of. But cancer lurked. Cancer that metastasized in the liver killed my father (he was 80), and there are other cancers in my family history. Plus, it didn't seem like there was much you could do about preventing its onset, with the possible exception of lung cancer—see Chapter 1—and I was not a smoker.

Since my father's troubles started in the colon, I had been enduring the every-five-years-or-so colonoscopy for quite a while. It's been uneventful outside of the residual effect that I can no longer quaff orange Gatorade, the drink I choose to accompany that horrible liquid involved with the bowel prep.

I remember that my father had urinary difficulties that stemmed from an enlarged prostate, but I had no idea how one combated that, and my father and I were never much for protracted discussions of any kind, far less ones of a sensitive medical nature.

Dr. Manley started me on prostate-specific antigen (PSA) screening when I was in my mid-40s, but I couldn't have told you what the letters stood for, what the numbers meant, or even exactly what the hell it was screening for. "Let's see, your blood work's good, cholesterol's under control, PSA's under 2 . . ." Dr. Manley would intone, and I would nod like a dope and feel like I just passed a test in a course I hadn't known I was taking.

What finally got my attention about the PSA level was the brave but ultimately futile struggle that a friend of mine named George Yasso had with prostate cancer. George was diagnosed with metastatic prostate disease in 2001 and never got better (see Chapter 15 for his story). After George got sick, I still didn't understand the inner workings of PSA, but its measurement started to feel more real.

Speaking of feeling real, having a digital rectal examination (DRE) was my least favorite occasion of the year. I began thinking about it a full month before Dr. Manley's invading finger approached my anus. He could give me an armful of shots with Brobdingnagian needles and it wouldn't bother me, but the thought of a single digit inserted into a very private space put me off my game. I was pondering going to the David Cronenberg movie *Cosmopolis* until I learned that the character played by Robert "Twilight" Pattinson receives a DRE in the backseat of his limo. That's not all he receives back there apparently, but it was enough to keep me away.

My wife rolled her eyes when I complained about the DRE, reminding me that the medical indignities routinely heaped upon the female—and beginning at a younger age—are far worse. Message received, but not helpful. My blood pressure would jump 20 points before the exam, and I always made some joking attempt to discourage the doctor from performing it.

"I felt my prostate just this morning, Doc," I'd say, "and it was fine."

"Terrific," he'd answer, diabolically wiggling his fingers into a rubber glove. "Now bend over and put your hands on the side of the table. You're going to feel a slight pressure and the need to urinate."

When a physician performs the exam, he or she feels the peripheral zone of the prostate, which constitutes about 65 to 70 percent of the gland's total area. (The other two zones are the central, with 20 to 25 percent, and the transition, with 5 to 10 percent of the total area.) I asked Dr. Manley how a doctor learns to perform a DRE. "Usually when a man is being prepped for surgery," he said. "Residents do it under the guidance of a urologist while the man is asleep. Bringing seven residents into an office to do a DRE on one guy doesn't work too well."

To perform the exam, a physician runs his finger along the surface of the prostate from front to back. "Before you do it you need to visualize the prostate, what a normal one would feel like," said Dr. Manley. "And like everything else in medicine, you have to see a lot of normals to appreciate the abnormal."

And how might it be abnormal?

"The consistency, the shape, the size, all of those things," said Dr. Manley. "I have felt what turned out to be cancer many times. It might feel like a pebble under the skin. Or it might just feel rough, bumpy.

"Now, if something is 'abnormal,' that doesn't mean a man has cancer. I've felt a bump and it turned out to be a calcium deposit. A family practitioner should never pronounce a man to have prostate cancer based on a physical exam. Our job is to determine, by the DRE and the PSA, if there's reason to suggest seeing a urologist."

Dr. Manley had never digitally detected anything unusual about my prostate, other than that it was "smallish," which is medically comforting but not necessarily a word that a male of any age wants to hear in relation to his reproductive system. But during my July 2011 physical, Dr. Manley expressed concern about my blood work.

"Your PSA is 3.8," he said. "That's not overly high, but the concern is how it has steadily risen."

My PSA was 1.4 in 2007, 1.7 in both 2008 and 2009, 2.23 in 2010, and now it was 3.888. There is some dispute about the meaningfulness of PSA "velocity"—the rate at which it rises—but to the doctors at Johns Hopkins, who have done much research on it, velocity is highly significant. "Your PSA should not go up more than 0.4 per year," says Dr. Patrick Walsh of Johns Hopkins.

Dr. Manley recognized mine as a fairly significant bounce and dropped a minor bomb.

"I think you should get a prostate biopsy," he said.

I suspect that everyone has a few clusters of words that can turn them into Jell-O. Perhaps it's "creamed chip beef on toast." Or "ringworm epidemic." Or "they just created a 24-hour Newt Gingrich channel." For me, "get a prostate biopsy" was right up there. That's because years earlier, a college buddy, Mike Steinhilber, described his biopsy thusly: "They stick a needle in your butt and then it feels like they open up a beach chair." A writer acquaintance of mine, Jeff Jarvis, best known for the book *Public Parts* and himself a member of the Prostate Cancer Club (see Chapter 15), has a different description of the biopsy, which typically involves taking about a dozen samples. "It's like shooting harpoons up your ass," says Jarvis.

Another college friend, Keith Van Arsdalen, MD, is a respected urological surgeon at the University of Pennsylvania, so I sent him my records. He agreed that a biopsy was warranted.

"Can you be asleep for this procedure, Keith?" I asked. "Or maybe half dead? See, Steiny told me once"—Mike and Keith are friends, also—and I went on to relate the beach-chair metaphor.

"Well, I don't think it's that bad," Keith said. "But it's uncomfortable, and, yes, more and more men are being put to sleep for the procedure." Thankfully, he didn't add, "Especially if they're wimps." He said that I would have to come to the hospital for routine testing before the procedure because it involves the use of anesthesia.

I talked it over with my wife and decided I would go ahead with it. I trusted both Dr. Manley and Keith to dispense sound medical advice. "There's no rush," said Keith. "We'll do it in September." That way, I could enjoy a few more weeks of relaxation while thinking about a needle being shoved into my rectum and the possibility that I might have cancer. Hell, golf is bad enough.

So there it was on the calendar for September 7, 2011: "prostate biopsy."

It was about then that I began hearing the news that I might be nuts to be scheduling a biopsy, and, furthermore, that I should not have even gotten a PSA test. I was confused, and I was not alone.

Thus began a journey to parse what seems to be a disturbing reality with a confounding suggestion.

Some 28,000 men per year will die of prostate cancer.

But we should pretty much ignore it.

Huh?

CHAPTER 4

... In which the author, blissfully unconscious, gets his biopsy and feels confident, but soon gets a sobering phone call

A FEW DAYS BEFORE MY BIOPSY, I was playing golf with a friend of mine, Marc Hellman, who wanted to know if I had ejaculated in the hours preceding the PSA test that had read 3.8.

"You won't believe this, Marc, but I don't keep a calendar of those things," I said.

"Because I heard that ejaculation can elevate the PSA," he said. Marc himself had gotten a negative biopsy after a higher-than-normal PSA reading. The same thing had happened to two other friends, and all of them thought that ejaculating before the blood test might've raised their numbers.

There have been studies testing this theory, and the conclusion seems to be that it might raise the PSA number, particularly if the blood is drawn within 24 to 48 hours of ejaculating, but both the rise and the proportion of men affected are small.

I didn't remember whether I had ejaculated, but at any rate I started to become convinced that, whatever the reason for my PSA rise, I would not be strolling down Prostate Pathway. I did not have cancer. That was my mind-set.

Biopsy day begins the way all depressing days should begin: with an enema, one of those Fleet jobs that is supposedly easy to self-administer. In my case, though, it required summoning my wife, whose "for better or worse" vows were severely tested.

I trust it is clear by now that when I did not enter the field of medicine, it was not a loss for the world at large.

Before the biopsy at Penn began, there was so much attendant rigmarole—insertion of the IV, conversation with the anesthesiologist, a run through the risk checklist, which includes, of course, death—that I began to feel guilty about getting put to sleep. Plus, the whole thing took so much time, and impatience is the clear leader in my long list of undesirable qualities. Had I submitted to the manly way of doing things, they would've sat me down, told me to bite on a towel like in an old Western, opened up that beach chair inside of me, harpooned away, and shoved me out the door.

I got wheeled into the OR, the guilt continuing. The small army of attendants suggested I was about to undergo a heart transplant. The room was cold and huge.

"You sure you need to do all this, Keith?" I said when he entered.

"It's what we do when there's anesthesia involved," he said.

Guilt. And then sleep. And then I was back where I started, my wife sitting near me reading the *Philadelphia Inquirer*.

"Your prostate is small, which is good," Keith said when he came in. "Everything looked fine, but you can't tell by a biopsy. Take care and I'll call you when I get the results. Remember—no driving. Donna drives home. Even if you feel fine, you had anesthesia."

It had been a long day, but I was relieved. We sat in the hospital cafeteria and I began deconstructing Keith's words like an amateur Kremlinologist. "Everything looked good." "Your prostate is small."

"I don't think I have prostate cancer," I said.

"I don't, either," Donna said.

About 25 to 35 percent of men who get biopsied for prostate cancer come up positive. Some studies suggest that the number is even lower if the PSA was below 4, and mine was 3.8.

The percentages were with me.

Then we drove to Vermont to see our son, who teaches at Middlebury College. I climbed into the driver's seat as my wife glared at me.

"You're not supposed to be driving," she said.

"Hey," I said. "I feel fine."

And that was that. I knew that the needle had gone into my prostate because I peed blood for a few days and it remained in my ejaculate for a while, too. But other than time wasted, the scoreboard read, as I saw it: one biopsy, no pain (not even soreness), no fuss, no muss, no cancer.

ABOUT 10 DAYS LATER my wife and I were driving home from the beach when Keith called me on my cell.

"I have good news and bad news," he said.

The first time I heard that line was on an episode of *Hogan's Heroes*, an inane 1960s sitcom that had had its moments.

"I have good news and bad news," Colonel Klink, the German commander, told the Americans.

"What's the bad news?" asked Hogan.

"You are to be shot at sunrise" was the answer.

"What could possibly be the good news?" Hogan asked.

"They have decided not to drag your body through the streets" was the answer.

I pulled over to the shoulder of the Garden State Parkway.

"The report shows cancer in 2 of the 12 sections we biopsied," Keith said.

And the good news? They will not be dragging my walnut-sized prostate through the streets?

"It's a very low level of cancer," Keith said. "It's manageable. We'll take care of this."

"So what's the next step?" I asked.

"Well, our procedure is to do an MRI with an anal probe," he said. "We do that so that—"

"Excuse me, Keith," I said. "Did you say 'anal probe'? I went to sleep for a biopsy and you're going to put an anal probe in me? I thought that's what happens to people who get kidnapped by aliens."

Keith explained that they do the probe MRI for several reasons.

- **Perhaps the cancer will be visible in the image (though probably not with a low level of cancer).**

- **The MRI produces a picture of the nearby lymph nodes; if cancer is suspected there, the nodes are biopsied, and chances are the prostate will not be removed if the cancer has spread. (Again, that would be an unlikely outcome given the low level of cancer in my prostate.)**

- **An MRI also provides an image that, if necessary, can be compared to later images to show any movement of the cancer or changes in other organs.**

Keith allowed that it was probably examination overkill, a CYA (cover your ass) move (or, in this case, a cover-*my*-ass move) that drives up the cost of medical care but helps protect doctors against liability and might be revelatory.

"Look, with cancer, you never know," he said.

It was a phrase I would hear, and utter myself, many times over the next year. "The golden rule of prostate cancer is," reads a maxim on the You Are Not Alone Now Web site devoted to supporting men with prostate cancer (yananow.org), "there are no rules."

And so I had cancer. Not much of it, but cancer nevertheless. Something happens to you then. You're a cancer victim, no matter what your level of victimhood. You have the Big C. You have, as Siddhartha Mukherjee's best-selling book put it, the Emperor of All Maladies. I didn't feel shock, outrage, or depression. I didn't declare war on the cosmos. I didn't mark down the date and only remember it now (September 16, 2011) because I had to go through my records as I researched this book. I knew I shouldn't even complain about it. Young kids get leukemia. Young kids die of brain tumors.

But I had cancer. I was one of Those People.

It's funny, but at the same time my wife and I turned to each other and said, "Let's not tell the kids." Because there's no easy way to tell somebody you have cancer. It always sounds bad, even if it isn't.

THE FIRST TIME I HAD AN MRI, about 20 years ago, I quite literally didn't know what I was getting into. They laid me on a hard board, slid me into an airless tube, put on elevator music that would've offended a lobotomy casualty, and told me to lie as still as a mummy for 40 minutes.

"Excuse me," I yelled about two minutes into the procedure, "but get me the hell outta here!"

They reluctantly pulled me out, no doubt calculating the minutes lost to the bottom line. I asked them to change the sound track to Van Morrison—I think they put on Van Cliburn, but it was an upgrade— took a couple of deep breaths and somehow endured the procedure in a cold sweat.

So needless to say I am not a fan of MRIs, never mind those accompanied by an anal probe. I have subsequently seen ads for MRIs that "eliminate the need for prostate anal probes." Keep that in mind if an anal probe is in your future.

Once I was on the table, though, the anal probe wasn't that bad. It was uncomfortable going in, but I grew accustomed to it. (Then again, one grows accustomed to acid reflux.) As for the MRI—what can I tell you? Come up with your own system for passing the time. My friend Bob Fink suggested playing an imaginary round of golf, shot by shot, to pass the time. I tried that, got to the fifth hole at the Architects Golf Club's course in Phillipsburg, New Jersey, yanked my drive into the weeds, and mentally walked off the course. I decided to simply count. They had said 40 minutes, and it was over in 30.

By now it was early October, and the flood of stories about abstaining from PSAs had only intensified. My cancer would not have been found if my family physician hadn't learned about my elevated number. Didn't that matter? Weren't people dying from this disease? Would I truly have been better off not knowing, which seems to go against every medical tenet, not to mention plain logic?

And, moreover, what was I going to do about it?

CHAPTER 5

... In which the author talks to a real person from the controversial USPSTF and wades into the murky waters of prostate cancer politics

THE *NEW YORK TIMES,* in my opinion the greatest newspaper there ever was and probably ever will be, had leapt with both feet, or whatever appendage the Old Gray Lady is standing on these days, into covering prostate cancer. As I pondered the fact that I had prostate cancer, hardly a day went by, it seemed, when there was not an article about the subject in the Paper of Record. And the relentless drumbeat came with a consistent admonition:

Do not get a PSA test.

What? My test and subsequent biopsy had already determined that I had cancer, albeit at a low volume, and now I'm supposed to accept that I shouldn't have been tested in the first place?

Since I have spent my entire adult life in journalism, I am not inclined to buy into conspiracy theories about my business. It is my experience that we in the media are far too disorganized and internally argumentative to launch fusillades against specific targets. But while the *Times*'s stories on prostate cancer were based on reporting—i.e., they quoted medical sources and did not editorialize—it seemed to this interested prostate observer that they went overly heavy on the warnings against getting tested.

To be fair, the prostate wasn't the *Times*'s only antitesting target. In the summer of 2012 Elisabeth Rosenthal, an environmental reporter and medical doctor, wrote an opinion piece suggesting that yearly physicals were a waste of time, too. So maybe there was a general *Times* jeremiad against standardized medical testing of all kinds.

But prostate patter clearly predominated, and the warnings against testing were attributed, by and large, to the US Preventive Services Task Force (USPSTF). The first thing I would say about this group is that it has an overly complicated name. I memorized all of its adjectives and nouns, but I keep putting them in different places: The US Services Task Force on Prevention. The US Task Force on Preventive Services. The US Preventive Task Force Service. Plus, I think the longer "Preventative" sounds more natural than "Preventive," though either, according to the dictionary, is acceptable as an adjective. However, "preventative" can also be a noun, as in "Crackers are a preventative for a hangover" (which has not been proven to my satisfaction).

But on one point the 16 volunteers making up the USPSTF made itself clear: Routine PSA testing is not a preventive for prostate cancer. In fact, the panel believes that it is quite the opposite.

I should make one point at the outset: The USPSTF is not the government "death panel" so colorfully described by Sarah Palin, she of the enlightened societal discourse. That is the Independent Payment Advisory Board (IPAB), which is charged with helping to reduce the rate of growth in Medicare spending, a purported bipartisan objective that has not turned out that way. But there's no doubt that under President Obama's Affordable Care Act, the USPSTF and the IPAB are at the very least first cousins.

The USPSTF is, according to its Web site, "an independent panel of non-Federal experts in prevention and evidence-based medicine and is composed of primary care providers (such as internists, pediatricians, family physicians, gynecologists/obstetricians, nurses, and health behavior specialists)." You will notice that "non-Federal" appears early; the organization wants to make it clear that it is not—technically—a federal agency.

USPSTF's charge is to conduct "scientific evidence reviews of a broad range of clinical preventive health care services (such as screening, counseling, and preventive medications) and [develop] recommendations for primary care clinicians and health systems."

So what does all that mean?

First, it is disingenuous of the organization to distance itself completely from Washington, DC. It is under contract to the Agency for Healthcare Research and Quality (AHRQ), which is part of the US Department of Health and Human Services—which the last time I checked was part of the federal government. The 16 USPSTF members, in fact, are appointed by the AHRQ's director.

Second, it is correct that the panel is not an enforcement agency and can only make recommendations. It does so by assigning letter grades to various medical procedures. Those grades are A, B, C, and D, just like in school, and also I, which means the USPSTF has "insufficient evidence" to recommend for or against the procedure. The target audience for the USPSTF is not specialists, but rather family practitioners.

At its most altruistic, then, its goal is to establish best practices within all branches of medicine and to establish them at the "entry level" for patients seeking care—primary care physicians. The USPSTF's official position is that it does not consider cost when analyzing the utility of preventive services. David Katz, MD, the director of the Yale-Griffin Prevention Research Center, wrote on *Huffington Post* on May 29, 2012, that the USPSTF "can certainly be trusted." He continued, "A unique feature of this group is that while they do have skin in the game of evidence-based recommendations, they have no skin in the game of clinical care that ensues. In other words, members of the task force don't lose or win if we do, or don't, screen for prostate cancer. They have no stake in the use of any particular test or technology."

But it simply strains credulity that the panel does not consider cost, particularly in our current political and fiscal environment. "Best practices" doesn't necessarily mean "cheapest," but it's not stretching the point to say that it means "best bang for the buck."

"The object of the task force, ostensibly, is to save lives," says Keith Van Arsdalen, my urologist, "but it's really to save money. So if you want to save money, and you can do 3 PSAs as opposed to doing 30 PSAs, you'll save a truckload."

The USPSTF has been around for nearly three decades, but no one paid much attention to it until 2009, when it made headlines by taking on the efficacy of mammograms with the recommendation that women between the ages of 50 and 74 get a mammogram every other year, but women younger than 50 get mammograms only when individual circumstances warrant.

From a public relations standpoint, that proclamation did not quite rise to the level of advocating the clubbing of baby seals, but it came close. After making the breast cancer recommendation, the USPSTF also recommended that electrocardiograms, whether done at rest or during a stress test, not be performed on people who have no known risks or symptoms of heart disease, such as shortness of breath and chest pains. Heart disease is perhaps the overarching issue in health care, yet you heard zilch about that recommendation. The message: Nothing in our health care universe engenders the pink-ribboned passion of breast cancer.

After the mammography recommendation was made public, criticism came from everywhere—congresspeople, medical professionals, advocates, and, most fervently, survivors whose cancer had been detected by a routine mammogram. Months of public wrangling about mammograms ensued, during which the word "ta-tas" was elevated to holy writ. The embattled USPSTF tried to make the case that, while its message got bungled, its methodology was solid. It was essentially a "communication problem," as it was put to me, which is what President Obama said was the primary reason for the negative reaction to the Affordable Care Act.

Clearly, one should not mess with the breast, and, after the outcry, the USPSTF walked back its recommendation. It now "recommends screening mammography, with or without clinical breast examination, every 1–2 years for women aged 40 and older." It gave that procedure a B rating, which means there is "moderate certainty" that the net benefit is "moderate to substantial" for women. Can you imagine how many meetings it took to come up with that wording?

An A rating means that the USPSTF "recommends" that clinicians provide the service to eligible patients because its net benefit is "substantial." Medicare is required to pay for a mammogram because it is a "recommended" procedure (and because Congress said it had to in a 1990 law). As for private insurers, it is reasonable to assume that they will continue to pay for most A- and B-rated tests, though making assumptions about what insurance companies will do is surely a fool's game.

On C ratings, the USPSTF drops back to punt by saying that it "makes no recommendation for or against routine provision of the service" if the doctor feels it's needed and the patient wants it. It's equally safe to assume that many insurers will not pay for Cs.

Which brings us to the USPSTF's current whipping boy—the PSA test. I'll say this for the panel: It doesn't shrink from controversy. Three years after the mammogram kerfuffle subsided, the organization doubled down by giving PSA screening a D. From a classroom perspective, the mammogram may not have been in the highest reading group, but it received a gold star or two along the way; the PSA test, by contrast, was ordered to stand in the corner and miss recess.

D ratings carry this declaration: "The USPSTF recommends *against* the service. There is moderate or high certainty that the service has no benefit or that the harms outweigh the benefits." (Emphasis mine.)

However under the radar prostate cancer had been flying at the time, it now became a polestar.

Whatever one thinks of the panel, it is unquestionably an organization under perpetual siege, rather like the reservations staff at a trendy New York City restaurant. I called the USPSTF and was referred to Michael LeFevre, MD, one of the Chosen 16. He is a professor in the Department of Family and Community Medicine at the University of Missouri and the co–vice chair of the USPSTF.

Dr. LeFevre was honest enough to clarify the federal connection upfront. "We are not federal employees," he said without my asking. "But when I fly to Washington for a conference, they feed me. And I get a $150 stipend for a two-day conference."

I wondered, first of all, if the PSA denouncement had produced anything like the hubbub caused by the mammogram recommendation.

"The mammogram blowback was tremendous, very, very intense," said Dr. LeFevre. "I would contrast the blowback for the PSA as much more muted. And the blowback came largely from two camps— urologists and prostate cancer survivors."

One thing was certain right away—"blowback" was the chosen word for "criticism." I'm not sure how to measure "muted." My surgeon, Dr. Lee, heard that the blowback totaled 20,000 comments, "95 percent of them negative." For the record, the official response from the American Urological Association (AUA) went like this: "[We are] outraged at the USPSTF's failure to amend its recommendations on prostate cancer testing to more adequately reflect the benefits of the [PSA] test in the diagnosis of prostate cancer."

The urologists were also offended that they were not represented (they still aren't) on the panel, William Catalona, MD, director of the Clinical Prostate Cancer Program at Northwestern University and a towering figure in the urological world, told me in an interview. No specialist likes a nonspecialist telling him or her what to do, and "they were completely devoid of cancer study expertise." Further, urologists resented the attention that was given to the panel. The AUA might have been an amateur athletic organization for all the general public knew, but the USPSTF was suddenly the darling of the *New York Times*.

"They are so cocky and so convinced that they're correct," says Dr. Walsh, "that nothing would change their mind." Adds Dr. Lee, who is not much given to sarcasm, "The guys from this panel are basically on tour."

Such complaints, however, are not specific to urology; the Chosen 16 are experts in biostatistics and research, not individual medical disciplines. "It would simply be impossible to have specialists for 50 different specialties," says Dr. LeFevre. "We are experts in prevention, evidence-based medicine. We make no apologies for that."

Dr. LeFevre says that urologists were consulted in the early stages of the panel's investigation. "We started by formulating a research plan," says Dr. LeFevre. "We said to ourselves, 'What questions do we need to be answered?' and we laid out those questions. 'Are these the right questions? Are these the right studies to look at? Is this a fair review? Did we miss studies? Did we misinterpret anything?' What we do is evidence-based procedure."

Again, there is disagreement about how much consultation went on. They didn't talk to either Dr. Walsh or Dr. Catalona, the men say, which is roughly like icing out Jonas Salk on a polio issue—Dr. Walsh is arguably the most important person in the history of prostate cancer treatment, and Dr. Catalona is the man most responsible for using PSA to screen for prostate cancer. There is absolutely no doubt that both doctors would've argued against scrapping the PSA test. But shouldn't the USPSTF have at least asked for their input, if only to defuse criticism that it hadn't?

In formulating its recommendations against PSA testing, the USPSTF studied the results of two major trials: the US PLCO (Prostate, Lung, Colorectal, and Ovarian) Cancer Screening Trial and the ERSPC (European Randomized Study of Screening for Prostate Cancer). According to the panel, the US trial "did not demonstrate any prostate cancer mortality reduction" and the European trial "found a reduction in prostate cancer deaths of approximately 1 death per 1,000 men screened in a subgroup of men aged 55 to 69 years."

Dr. Walsh, Dr. Catalona, and scores of others say that the USPSTF misinterpreted the data.

"I'm sure they're good people," says Dr. Walsh, "but the problem is they don't know anything about prostate cancer. They relied on 10-year survival, but there is now a very good study from Scandinavia that is a 30-year follow-up. At 9 years, yes, the risk of death from prostate cancer is negligible, but at 15 years and beyond it's three times higher. It's really pathetic what they've done."

Understand that this is heavy-duty, graduate-level statistical stuff, much of it beyond the scope of this book. But if you're the kind of person who likes to climb into bed with a book on, say, binomial coefficients in Pascal's triangle, feel free to have at it. Links to the studies are furnished in the Sources and Resources section of this book, and other summations and arguments for and against the conclusions about both trials are readily available on the Internet.

The key thing to remember is that the USPSTF's interpretation was that PSA screening not only did not save lives across the population, but also caused harm. According to the panel, that harm could come from:

- **Serious infection from the prostate biopsy**
- **Serious risks posed by the intervention, whether surgical or radiological**
- **Permanent side effects in the form of erectile dysfunction and urinary incontinence in the event of unnecessary treatment**

Without exactly smothering the panel with wet kisses, the American Cancer Society, or at least the most influential member of it, Otis Brawley, MD, is clearly on the side of the USPSTF. The society's chief medical officer and a professor at Emory University, Dr. Brawley wrote a 2012 book called *How We Do Harm: A Doctor Breaks Ranks about Being Sick in America* (coauthored with Paul Goldberg, a longtime muckraker in the cancer world) that is primarily about the perils of overtreatment. But when Dr. Brawley is presented as antiscreening, he demurs and says, rather, that he advocates telling men the whole prostate story instead of just ordering up a PSA test. "It's a shame when a man is screened for prostate cancer and not told that his cigarette smoking is more likely to kill him than prostate cancer," Dr. Brawley told the magazine *Atlanta* in February 2012.

That makes absolute sense. But it's impossible to wade through the corporate speak and get this nation's most influential cancer spokesman to take a clear position on the USPSTF recommendation. In an opinion piece for CNN.com in May 2012, Dr. Brawley wrote that "the task force's methods are notable for their scientific rigor," and "for two decades, mass PSA-based prostate cancer screening was done in this country without direct clinical evidence showing that it was beneficial to patients." But he won't directly say that he agrees with the USPSTF. He writes that he hopes "that this new recommendation will put an end to mass screening."

But is Dr. Brawley against all screening, which is the USPSTF's message? Does he agree with the D recommendation that PSA screening is harmful? That much isn't clear. (I reached out to Dr. Brawley for a comment, but did not hear back.)

As with breast cancer, much of the hue and cry against the recommendation came not just from specialists, but also from men who had survived prostate cancer. They included Representative John Barrow, a Democrat from Georgia, who cosponsored House Resolution 5998, the USPSTF Transparency and Accountability Act of 2012. It would mandate that the USPSTF consult more closely with specialists and is still pending at this writing.

Indeed, the screening controversy has never been far from politics, not in an environment in which "Obamacare" was turned into a four-letter word throughout the endless 2012 election cycle. One of the architects of the Affordable Care Act was Ezekiel Emanuel, MD, brother of Rahm Emanuel, Obama's former chief of staff. Dr. Emanuel, now the chair of the Department of Medical Ethics and Health Policy at the University of Pennsylvania's Perelman School of Medicine, has campaigned vigorously against what he considers needless medical procedures, and he was cast as one of the chief "death panel" villains.

Many others have politicized the issue. Paul Hsieh, MD, cofounder of Freedom and Individual Rights in Medicine, wrote an opinion piece that ran on *Forbes* magazine's Web site on July 5, 2012, under the headline: "Is President Obama's Prostate Gland More Important Than Yours?" He wrote, accurately, that Obama, upon turning 50, had requested and received a PSA test. Wrote Dr. Hsieh: "When President Obama had his routine physical last year, he enjoyed the freedom to consult with his doctors, weigh the pros and cons of PSA testing, and decide for himself what was in his best medical interest. But under

ObamaCare, the President will not allow you that same freedom. Instead, the federal government will decide for you."

At this writing, Medicare is still covering PSA screening despite its D rating. But it is not unreasonable to conclude that that might change. And it is certainly reasonable to surmise that private insurers will stop paying for screenings that have been bashed by a review board with government ties. Here's more ammunition justifying not paying: The American Academy of Family Physicians (AAFP) has adopted the panel's recommendation against screening.

Although all the talk from the Right about "death panels" has a hysterical tone to it, the issue raised by Dr. Hsieh, who is no fan of the president, is legitimate. It also highlights the fact that this controversy, adjudged from a political perspective, is at once predictable and incongruous.

The predictable: Democrats are trying to force-feed government down our throats with recommendations that are de facto mandates, while Republicans are all for individual freedom, a free-flowing discussion between doctor and patient.

The incongruous: Democrats are trying to cut needless costs that are strangling our health care system, while Republicans are insisting upon unnecessary tests that drive up our health care debt.

Oh, what a tangled web that won't get untangled soon. Researchers continue to come up with drugs (three new ones are sipuleucel-T [Provenge], abiraterone acetate [Zytiga], and cabazitaxel [Jevtana]) that extend the lives of prostate cancer patients. They are all expensive and they all raise the age-old question of whether they are worth the cost of extending life. What is really needed is a test administered in the early stages of prostate cancer that would better predict its course.

Clearly, the civil war will go on. "Outside of urology, there has been support for the USPSTF," says Sloan-Kettering's Peter Bach, who is well known in the field of medical research. "I think [the recommendation against screening] is a direction. We have a long history in health care of adopting technologies and using them more broadly than what they were originally designed for."

But remember that the USPSTF's target is family practitioners, and they have by no means embraced the recommendation, the position of the AAFP notwithstanding. James Manley, my doctor, says he is squarely against the USPSTF's decision and will continue to suggest that most of his patients, even those as young as 40, get PSA screening annually. And you must understand how strongly urologists stand against the recommendation. Jerry Blaivas, MD, a celebrated New York City urologist, is not in favor of PSA screening (you'll find more on his views in Chapter 13), yet he considers the USPSTF meddlesome. "I don't mind thoughtful panels or even a recommendation," says Dr. Blaivas. "But I am utterly opposed to a government mandate if that's what this comes to."

So where did all of that leave a man who had already gotten a biopsy because of an elevated PSA? Should I have found a time machine and returned to cancel out all my previous PSA readings?

Here's a better question: Where did the PSA test come from? And another: Does it tell us anything useful?

CHAPTER 6

...In which the author finds out what the inventor of the PSA test has to say

IN THE MARCH 10, 2010, EDITION of the *New York Times*, an opinion piece written by Richard Ablin, PhD, appeared under the headline "The Great Prostate Mistake." Dr. Ablin identified himself as the discoverer of PSA, described the test as "hardly more effective than a coin toss," and concluded, "I never dreamed that my discovery four decades ago would lead to such a profit-driven public health disaster."

The column drew widespread attention. To state the obvious, those who agreed generally with the USPSTF that prostate testing was overdone and harmful applauded the piece, while those in the urological establishment and elsewhere who favored PSA testing criticized it. The latter group also included many who believed that Dr. Ablin oversold his urological credentials. Certainly the *Times* did in identifying him as the inventor of the PSA test, something the newspaper later retracted.

Yes, like almost everything else in the prostate cancer world, the identification of the prostate-specific antigen and the origin of the test most often used to measure the amount of PSA in a man's blood are steeped in controversy. Before delving into that, though, some basics are necessary.

An antigen is a substance that causes the immune system to produce one or more antibodies against it. So the prostate-specific antigen is exactly what its name indicates: an antigen produced by the prostate. That antigen's role is to liquefy semen so the sperm in the ejaculate are able to swim. Under normal conditions PSA is secreted and disposed of through tiny ducts in the prostate, but prostate cancer doesn't have a working ductal system. As Dr. Walsh explains it, its ducts are "blind, dead-end streets." So rather than drain into the urethra, PSA builds up, leaks out of the prostate, and shows up in the bloodstream, where it can be measured as a marker for cancer.

According to Dr. William Catalona, who has done research into the origins of PSA and the PSA test, the earliest report on the properties of antigens in the prostate was by Iowa urologist Rubin Flocks in 1960. In the mid-1960s, a Japanese forensic scientist, Mitsuwo Hara, partially characterized and reported on a protein similar to PSA. According to Dr. Catalona, Hara called it "gamma-seminoprotein" and suggested its possible value as forensic evidence in rape cases.

Dr. Ablin was next. On the Web site of the Robert Benjamin Ablin Foundation for Cancer Research, which Dr. Ablin founded in memory of his father, who died of metastatic prostate cancer, it is written: "Dr. Richard J. Ablin and his research team discovered antigens of the human prostate, including prostate tissue-specific antigen, that later became known as PSA."

At least a dozen interview subjects told me that this discovery was not significant, and that, at any rate, Dr. Ablin's work had nothing to do with the development of the PSA test, which was a task separate and distinct from that of antigen isolation. Clearly, I am not the one to judge whether or not his discovery was scientifically significant.

I reached out to Dr. Ablin, who is a professor of pathology at the University of Arizona, but was not granted an interview. "He is currently working on his own book, and I have advised him not to contribute to any other," said his literary agent from William Morris.

There is no doubt that credit for development of the PSA *test* belongs elsewhere, to a man and a team working at the Roswell Park Cancer Institute in downtown Buffalo, which once ranked right up there with the MD Anderson Cancer Center in Houston and Memorial Sloan-Kettering Cancer Center in New York City as a leading cancer research facility and teaching hospital. It was at Roswell in the 1970s that a Taiwanese native named T. Ming Chu, PhD, and his team of scientists and researchers created the test that launched a new age in prostate cancer detection and treatment.

Dr. Chu, a gentle, soft-spoken man in his mid-70s, has been retired for several years, though he remains a professor emeritus of cancer pathology and prevention at Roswell. He and his wife live in the Sandhills region of North Carolina but keep a home in Buffalo, which Dr. Chu visits frequently to fly-fish, his main hobby.

As Dr. Ablin was isolating his antigen, Dr. Chu, armed with a PhD in biochemistry from Pennsylvania State University and three years of post-doc study, arrived at Roswell Park. He received what he calls his "marching orders" from Gerald Murphy, MD, a famed urologist and the director at Roswell. "Dr. Murphy told me I could do whatever research I wanted as long as prostate cancer was part of it," Dr. Chu said.

At one time Dr. Chu also had National Institutes of Health grants to work on pancreatic and breast cancers, but, as long as Dr. Murphy was around, the prostate was not going to be shoved to the bottom of Chu's to-do list. The goal was clear: "I was to search for prostate cancer–specific or associate antigens," he says, "then develop a simple blood test."

Remember that PSA measurement had nothing to do with cancer *screening* back then; rather, it was a way to measure the volume of cancerous tissue in the prostate, which it does as nanograms of PSA per milliliter of blood. (A nanogram is one-billionth of a gram.)

It took Dr. Chu several years to get his team in place and secure the clinical support of urologists from around the country. There was no eureka moment, he says, it was more of "an accumulation of incremental results," but on a glorious day in 1979 Chu and his team isolated the antigen. They say it is wholly different from the antigen discovered by Dr. Ablin. Chu's team needed to do additional work to purify the antigen and, finally, to design the test, which happened in 1980.

Dr. Chu repeatedly emphasized that he did not make the discovery alone. During an interview at Roswell in November of 2012, he fired up his laptop and showed me a list of every researcher, scientist, and postdoc who worked on it with him, some two dozen names altogether.

But he also wants to make it just as clear that it is not Dr. Ablin who deserves credit.

"Dr. Ablin has never published a single peer-reviewed paper on the subject of PSA," says Dr. Chu. "I think he has some kind of complex."

The PSA work of Dr. Chu, who holds 11 other patents beside the PSA test, was widely recognized and applauded, and he remains a lofty personage in the urological world. Dr. Chu says that there is precious little difference in the test his team designed more than 30 years ago and the one being used today.

But from the beginning there was professional consternation about PSA test results, mainly because factors other than cancer—BPH and prostatitis (inflammation of the prostate), to name two—can elevate the PSA level. Somewhat sheepishly, the University of Rochester's Dr. Edward Messing remembers writing an early paper in which "I said we didn't know what to do with PSA." Says Dr. Van Arsdalen, my urologist: "Early on, everybody had a lot more hope that PSA would be better at differentiating cancer from noncancer. It's specific to the prostate, but it's not specific for prostate cancer." The best use for PSA when it first came out was as a marker for the recurrence of cancer, which remains a significant part of its employment today.

No one was—or is—more aware of PSA measurement's imperfection than Dr. Chu. "The biology of prostate cancer is very, very complex," says Dr. Chu. "It is a quite heterogeneous disease." He means that it is unpredictable, that the dreaded aggressive 20 percent just can't be easily characterized, and that a perfect blood test has yet to be designed. The joke in prostate cancer circles, in fact, is that "PSA" stands not for "prostate-specific antigen," but for "prostate-specific anxiety."

Over time, urologists learned more about PSA, how to use it, and when to use it, but the real revolution came when it became widely accepted as a screening test, not just as a marker of cancer volume (see the full story about that in the section on Dr. Catalona in Chapter 13). And eventually the PSA test affixed itself to the prostate cancer equation as closely as the mammogram did to breast cancer.

Even as the USPSTF recommends against the PSA test, there are ever more studies on and experiments using PSA, a constant tinkering.

Dr. Steven Kaplan, the New York-Presbyterian Hospital/Weill Cornell Medical College urologist, has led experiments that combine treatment with the BPH drugs finasteride (Proscar) or dutasteride (Avodart) with PSA readings over the course of a year in an effort to detect aggressive prostate cancer in men with high PSA levels who have had negative biopsies.

Men are increasingly getting the "free PSA test," which measures the amount of PSA that is not bound to other proteins in the blood; for reasons unknown, men with cancer have less free PSA than men who are cancer-free. There is also "PSA density" to calculate and consider. That number is arrived at by dividing the PSA reading by the volume of the prostate. The theory behind PSA density is that a man with benign disease would have a PSA density of about 10 percent and no higher than 15 percent of the weight of his prostate.

The "PCA3 test" is for men who have already had a negative biopsy but a question remains as to whether to do a repeat biopsy. One negative is that it involves an "attentive rectal exam," in which the doctor has to massage prostatic fluid into the urethra. (For pure amusement, that equates to repeatedly stapling your tongue.)

At this writing, the PCA3 test has just been approved by the FDA, as has the Prostate Health Index (PHI), which combines measurements of total PSA, free PSA, and a subcategory of free PSA called pro-PSA.

The search for a more perfect PSA test—or a more perfect replacement for it—will go on. But those discoveries will not be made by Dr. T. Ming Chu, who even hesitates to launch himself into the USPSTF recommendation debate. "I am not a urologist," he says, "and neither is Dr. Ablin. He is not involved in the screening and management of prostate cancer patients. He is a scientist and he should restrict debate and conversation to the scientific community."

But Dr. Chu has looked hard at the evidence used in making the USPSTF recommendation from the perspective of a researcher.

"Speaking strictly from a scientific point of view, the US trial that the panel used was mixed and contaminated," says Dr. Chu. "They based their findings upon a mixed bag of so-called clinical studies. They put oranges and apples together and compared them, so that the result would show no benefit from PSA testing."

You are welcome to weigh Dr. Chu's comments against the reality that he developed the PSA test. And you are welcome to note that PSA tests have become the low-hanging fruit of the medical-testing world. But in Dr. Chu I found a scrupulously honest man, one universally respected in his field.

"There is almost nothing perfect in the medical world," says Dr. Chu. "But I believe that PSA is as good a screening test for prostate cancer as the mammogram is for breast cancer."

CHAPTER 7

... In which the author consults with his urologist, visits a radiologist (just in case), decides against treatment, and opens himself up to second-guessing

AND SO IT CAME TIME FOR MY PROSTATE CANCER CONSULT with my urologist and college friend, Keith Van Arsdalen. Keith's resident entered the room first. He had the report from my biopsy and he sketched out the numbers.

The most basic way of determining the seriousness of prostate cancer is the Gleason score, a grading system that accounts for the differing patterns that prostate tumor cells take in relation to normal cells. My Gleason, the resident told me, was 3 + 3.

A 1 characterizes cells that are nearly normal, while a 5 represents cells that look completely different from normal prostate cells. The more different they are, the more like cancer they are, and consequently the more ominous they are.

The pathologist grades the two most common tumor patterns seen in the pieces removed from the prostate. So, with a 3, I was in the middle on both patterns. The 3 + 3 is the most common finding from a biopsy of this kind. My score is good news in a way, but as I would discover, it also makes the treatment decision particularly gnarly.

The Gleason should not be looked at like the PSA test's result, i.e., as a number subject to debate. Certainly there have been mistakes in pathology labs, but if your cancer is scored as, say, 5 + 5, it is an almost indisputable fact that you have aggressive prostate disease. It is not BPH and it is not prostatitis.

Since you're wondering, no, the score has nothing to do with the larger-than-life star of *The Honeymooners*. The Gleason is named for Donald Gleason, MD, PhD, the former chief pathologist at the Minneapolis Veterans Affairs Medical Center, where he developed the scoring system with other researchers in the 1960s and continued to refine it through the 1980s. When I visited Dr. Chu at Roswell Park, he showed me a slide from an original drawing that Dr. Gleason had made of cancers 1 through 5. It was riveting. The American Urological Association should make a T-shirt showing it. It looked like something that M. C. Escher would've produced after spending a couple of weeks as a Grateful Dead roadie. I studied my Gleason 3 for a long time; it was just starting to break out into a psychedelic pattern.

My biopsy also revealed cancer in 2 of 12 cores, one with 20 percent cancer, one with 5 percent. Not a large amount of cancer, but not negligible either.

The MRI and bone scan both showed no evidence that the cancer had spread. That was expected, but good news nevertheless.

All in all, if you're going to have cancer, I didn't have much to complain about. I had low-grade, localized prostate cancer.

Up to that point, my wife and I had not researched the subject all that deeply. Or, to clarify: I hadn't. Donna had done some homework, finding out the basics on prostatectomy (removal of the prostate and, thus, the cancer); radiation (from both internal and external sources, including brachytherapy, which means implanting cancer-fighting radioactive seeds in the prostate); and "watchful waiting," or, under its contemporary name, active surveillance. We were both intrigued by the latter. Maybe I wouldn't need an operation or radiation.

Then again, lurking in the back of my mind was the death from prostate cancer of my friend George Yasso. Cold logic demands that medical decisions be made on a personal basis, not on what happened to someone else. But it's human nature to consider what happened to someone else, especially someone close to you.

We also knew, in a general sense, the possible consequences of surgery. There could be impotence, temporary or permanent, as well as urinary-control issues, temporary or permanent. The former was more likely than the latter, but the research seemed to say there is no precise pre-intervention way to predict how either is going to come out. The surgeon can make an educated guess afterward based on how many nerves had to be cut during surgery, but he or she can't be absolutely sure how that will affect future sexual performance or urinary function.

There is in the prostate-discussion ether the idea that patients are not given enough information about these repercussions, i.e., that many men choose to have surgery or radiation and only later find out that they may never again have an erection. I've heard this from prostate cancer sufferers and read it on chat forums, and certainly the USPSTF believes that urologists are not always forthcoming about what surgery or radiation might do.

Frankly, I struggle to wrap my mind around that. There are good and bad urologists and good and bad communicators, no doubt about that, but does anyone these days go to a hospital for surgery or submit to more than a month of radiation therapy without glancing at the Internet? Most people check Yelp before shopping for applesauce.

Twenty years ago, even 10 years ago, information was harder to come by, and doctors dealt with mostly undereducated patients. But if you spend 30 seconds researching prostate cancer you will find "erectile dysfunction" and "incontinence" are the major connectives to intervention. In essence, they are the whole ball game. In pondering whether to have surgical or radiological intervention, a major part of the decision involves choosing whether you want to open Door Number 1 (ED), Door Number 2 (incontinence), or, perhaps, have both of them slam you in the face.

KEITH HAD LET US KNOW in his initial phone call that a treatment decision would not have to be made exigently or under duress. He had said that I should decide by early the next year. It was now October 6, about a month after my biopsy.

We brought up active surveillance with the resident and he seemed receptive to it. But he wasn't the boss.

Then Keith came in. One of life's adjustments—and maybe this is just for males—is reconciling an early friendship with an adult one. To an extent, you tend to eternally see the doctor who stands before you with a cancer report as the kid you got hammered with in college. It's easy to assess maturation and professional competence in yourself—or at least to imagine it—but it's sometimes difficult to do the same for old friends.

But that wasn't the case with Keith. He seemed adult and competent even when he was 18 (though, to be clear, I wouldn't have wanted him to do a DRE on me back in 1969). So there would be no mistrust of what he had to say. He was clearly my doctor, not my friend.

We shook hands, he pecked Donna on the cheek, and he got down to business.

"You have three basic courses of treatment," he began, pulling out a legal pad. "First, there is a way to treat this with what's called 'watchful waiting' or 'active surveillance.'"

My wife and I exchanged knowing glances. This seemed to be the way to go. No surgery, no radiation, no—

"So I would take that off the table," said Keith. I still have a mental picture of him literally crossing out the words "active surveillance."

Keith went on to discuss the other two possibilities—prostatectomy and radiation. He didn't advocate one over the other but allowed that he was a urologist, not a radiologist, so his inclination was for surgical intervention. He had performed many of those operations himself. "But I would recommend setting up an appointment with our radiology department so they can discuss those options," he said.

Keith also emphasized that, if I chose surgery, he would not do it. Unless a patient insisted otherwise, Keith and most other urologists in the University of Pennsylvania Health System refer cases like mine to Dr. David Lee, who performs prostatectomies with the da Vinci robot, a procedure that started to gain hold about 10 years ago. Keith has no experience with the robot; he trained using the original "open" method, which involves getting at the prostate via a "radical retropubic" incision down the lower abdomen or a "radical perineal" incision in the perineum, which is the area between the anus and the scrotum.

Before we left, I presented Keith with the question most commonly asked of urologists who are delivering cancer news.

"If I were your father instead of a friend, Keith," I said, "what would you advise?"

It's an unfair question, of course, but one that is asked all the time. John McHugh, MD, a prominent Georgia urologist, had an interesting response to this: "The irony of the question," writes Dr. McHugh in *The Decision*, a book about the treatment of and his experience with his own prostate cancer, "is that I am not a big fan of my father."

But I knew that Keith had a good relationship with his father.

"I'd tell him to get surgery," said Keith immediately. "But you have to make your own decision."

I tentatively offered that I had been thinking about active surveillance. Keith did not throw up his hands and collapse operatically on his desk. "It wouldn't be my first choice for you," he said. "But I don't think that it's a stupid decision. If I did, I would tell you." To be clear, Keith wanted me to have surgery, firmly believed that I should have surgery. But had I argued vociferously for active surveillance, which I wasn't prepared to do at the time, he wouldn't have stood in my way. With the level of cancer I had, the decision-making process, more than with most cancers, is in the hands of the patient. That's good, I suppose, but it's also confounding.

And so we left the consult aware of one salient fact: Figuring out what to do about my low level of prostate cancer would involve as much art as science. There were no absolutely correct answers and no absolutely wrong answers.

So that made it easier.

And harder.

"There are no rules!"

After our conference, I saw in a letter that Keith had written to my family physician: "I had a discussion with Jack regarding the options for localized prostate cancer in older men," it read.

Jesus, I not only had cancer but was also an "older man"? I had truly never considered that before.

A FEW WEEKS LATER I had a meeting with one of Penn's radiation oncologists, John Christodouleas, MD. He was glad that Keith had sent me. "Many patients never see a radiation oncologist because they get their information from the urologist," said Dr. C. "Keith did the right thing."

I liked Dr. C. despite the fact that, unexpectedly, he performed a digital rectal exam on me. I figured radiology guys adjusted beams, turned dials, and stayed the hell away from the nasty stuff, but it was SOP, Dr. C. said—a DRE helps him "score" the cancer. A Johns Hopkins radiologist was visiting Dr. C. that day, and he also performed a DRE. "On the way out," I said to Dr. C., "I'm going to ask the parking attendant if he wants to take a shot, make it a three-for-a-dollar day."

The fact that the doctors didn't feel anything, combined with my Gleason score and the results of the biopsy, made me a T1—"tumor present but not detectable by clinical exam or imaging." My cancer was more specifically a T1c, which meant that it was slightly worse than a T1a or a T1b but not as bad as a T2, which means that the tumor can be felt by clinical exam. A cancer graded a T3 means that it has escaped the prostate.

To explain the radiology option, Dr. C. sketched out a simple graph with "age" on one side, "intensity of side effects" on the other. In general—emphasis on "in general"—younger men do better with surgery and older men do better with radiation. "As patients get older," he said, "they don't tolerate surgery as well. They just don't recover the same way as younger patients. By contrast, with radiation, the longer you're alive the more at risk you are for secondary cancers caused by radiation. So we do not like to treat younger patients with radiation."

On Dr. C.'s graph, impotence and incontinence (the "side effects") crossed age somewhere around 65. Which means that theoretically, a person who is about 65 can expect similar outcomes from surgery and radiation. But that is a guess. An educated one, but a guess nevertheless. "What doctors don't agree on," said Dr. C., "is where these curves cross. Some people put it at 55, some people at 60, some people a little older. At 62, you're somewhere near that sweet spot."

Even men who have done sketchy research come to a radiology

session with this stark bit of information: If you have radiation and the cancer returns, neither further radiation nor surgical intervention will help you.

But Dr. C. says that is not quite true. "There are lots of things that can be done, including surgery," he said. "But it is true that many surgeons do not like to operate, and some will not operate, on men who have had radiation. The surgery is more complicated and the side effects are rougher on the patient."

The reason for that is the scar tissue that forms around the irradiated area. "Surgeons work easily when there are planes of dissection, and tissue can naturally separate along these planes," explained Dr. C. "After radiation, however, those planes of dissection fuse and it's much harder surgically. So it's not that you can't. It's that it's more complicated." And he added this: "The most important thing to remember is that meaningful reoccurrences of prostate cancer are extremely rare."

Translation: Dr. C. did not rule out radiation as a treatment modality simply because of that worst-case scenario of the cancer returning.

(I later asked my surgeon, Dr. Lee, about operating after radiation. He agreed it was more difficult, but doable. "I think the major concern is rectal injury during that type of surgery," said Dr. Lee. "Even if you sew it up correctly, guys can end up with really bad complications.")

I asked Dr. C. if patients make a choice based simply on "feel"—that art-trumping-science thing. He understood the question perfectly.

"If you had a bad experience in your family with radiation, you will probably say, 'I'm going to have surgery,'" he said. "Or surgery didn't work out for someone so you choose radiation. That is a perfectly fine reason for choosing one treatment or the other. As long as one understands the toxicity profile [his term for side effects], feeling one way or the other about a procedure is perfectly legitimate."

And halfway through Dr. C.'s discourse I knew how I felt. If I were going to get intervention, it would not be radiation. For these reasons:

1. I still didn't like that scenario by which the cancer
    could return and future options would become more
    difficult after radiation. I saw his point about surgery
    being more difficult but possible as a distinction
    without a difference.

2. I didn't feel like committing to the radiation routine,
    which involves 35 to 45 visits, usually on a 5-times-a-
    week schedule. If that's a silly reason for disliking it,
    well, that's okay, but it's my reason.

3. I am not scared of surgery, probably because I'm a
    veteran of it. Orthopedically, I've been through
    procedures on my neck, back, Achilles tendon, and both
    knees (arthroscopic), and for good measure, I had several
    inches of my colon snipped off because of diverticulitis.
    I came through everything just fine. Get in, get it done,
    move on: That is my philosophy.

4. As soon as I heard that the radiation beam passes
    close to the rectum—and Dr. C. was candid enough to
    admit that "rectal involvement" is a potential
    side effect, occurring in probably in 1 to 2 percent of
    cases and some say more—I crossed it off. I didn't want
    to make my rectum any part of this deal. Have I told
    you how much I hate digital rectal exams?

Take note that radiation is a main tool in cases where the cancer
has escaped the prostate; there is no value in removing the prostate
surgically if the cancer has spread. So I am not trashing radiation per
se. Plus, I interviewed urologists who greatly respect radiological
treatment. "Even for those of us who were trained as surgeons and

believe that surgery is how you get rid of cancer," says Pablo Torre, MD, a urologist at the Veterans Affairs Medical Center in New York City, "radiation therapy has come to the point where it's almost equivalent."

I will tell you negative things that other doctors had to say about radiation in Chapter 12, but they have more to do with philosophy and finances than they do with the procedure itself.

I can only tell you how I felt about it.

Then, too, at that time—early in the decision-making process—the fact that I put surgery ahead of radiation was academic.

"I feel pretty comfortable about active surveillance," I told my wife. She nodded her head. She did, too. Kind of. Sort of.

So I wrote an October 17, 2011, column for my local newspaper, the *Morning Call* in Allentown, Pennsylvania, talking mostly about how I now had the "It" disease, how the *New York Times* had weighed in on it, how urologists argued with task forces, how nobody was sure about what to do. And I informed the readers that I had chosen active surveillance.

Many of them called, e-mailed, or sent me a letter.

Some told me I was nuts.

THE MORNING CALL
OCTOBER 17, 2011

Weighing Pros, Cons of Cancer Treatment

While there's never a good time to get the Big C, I have to tell you: My timing on this one is pretty good. Since I was handed a diagnosis of prostate cancer a few weeks ago, people like me are all the rage. It's about time, too. None of my previous medical issues, most of an orthopedic nature, have [caught] fire with the public. And that diverticulitis thing? Trust me, nobody wants to talk about that, before, during or after lunch.

But once a few voices in the medical community suggested that prostate cancer is (a) overtested, (b) overdiagnosed, and (c) overtreated, we suddenly had a new It Disease. And I happen to be one of the new It Sufferers.

The slogan of The New York Times in recent weeks might as well have been: All the Prostate News That Fits, We Print. There have been segments on the nightly news, arguments in medical journals, spirited discussions on blogs. PC (does any disease more deserve its own acronym, even one that's already taken?) was even a topic in one of the 437 Republican presidential debates that have taken place recently. I don't have this nailed down, but I think that Newt Gingrich believes a cancerous prostate is a Democratic plot to institute death panels, while Herman Cain is positive that 9 percent of the prostate-cancer population should have surgery.

Anyway, my diagnosis and the concomitant avalanche of news articles have forced me to do something against my nature—careful research. (My preferred method of subject analysis had always been to ask my wife, "Would you Google that?" and wait for her answer between "Law and Order" reruns.)

But since I find myself in the medical spotlight, I'd like to share with you my thoughts on PC, with the hope that I can straighten out some of the inevitable confusion that has arisen out of this controversial recommendation. I submit that I deserve the stage, incidentally, having heard in recent weeks one of the most unsettling sentences in the English language: "Relax now, while we insert the anal probe, inflate the balloon and slide you into the MRI."

Just to give you the baseline information: I am a 62-year-old Caucasian male, in otherwise good health, aching knees notwithstanding. So here we go:

My family doctor suggested several months ago that I should see a urologist because my PSA level, while not alarmingly high, had risen.

Of course, the PSA test may not be reliable at all. But, lo and behold, this one did some good since a subsequent biopsy revealed cancer. But did I really need to know? Chances are, I'm going to die of something else since prostate cancer grows so slowly.

Still, I was glad to find out and also glad to hear that the amount of cancer is small and contained within the prostate. Good news. Then again, any cancer can spread and conceivably kill you. Bad news. But, remember . . . odds are, I'll die of something else. Well, that might be true if I was, say, 70. But 62 is too young to be sure about any kind of cancer.

I could get surgery and, chances are, the cancer will be gone forever. But surgery can bring about lingering problems of incontinence and erectile dysfunction. Yes, but these post-surgical effects are often not that bad.

But if they are, you're the guy trying to hide a box of adult Depends in his shopping cart under gallons of strawberry ice cream. Or you're the guy sitting in that ridiculous outdoor bathtub praying that things, you know, kick in before "The Daily Show" comes on.

Radiation is an excellent option. There are many variations to choose from. And if I had six years of medical school, maybe I could understand them all. But radiation is painless and, at my level of cancer, chances are the PC will be zapped forever. Except if it's not, radiation makes it almost impossible to go back in and get the cancer.

"Watchful waiting," also known as "active surveillance," is an option. True, as long as I can talk myself into forgetting that I have cancer. Which is kind of like forgetting that you've swallowed a javelin. With watchful waiting, I can keep an eye on things, get another biopsy in a year and more frequent PSA tests. Except that PSA tests might not be reliable. I believe this is where we all came in.

For the record, I have tentatively decided on a course of watchful waiting, which my wife and I are convinced is the correct decision.

Unless it's not.

CHAPTER 8

...In which the author gets a surprise at the Temple of Active Surveillance

THE STRATEGY OF NOT INTERVENING SURGICALLY or radiologically in prostate cancer started in Sweden as "watchful waiting." That seems logical because the whole strategy seems so positively Swedish. Find out you have an ominous-sounding disease, brood about it, pick up a Henning Mankell mystery about a grisly murder on the fjord, brood about it some more, get drunk on brännvin, brood about it some more....

I don't know if Sweden's socialized health care system had something to do with the movement toward watchful waiting, but watchful waiting—or "active surveillance," to use the latter-generation nomenclature—is based on sound medical evidence. To repeat—prostate cancer is a slow-growing cancer, and there is much evidence that many men who have it will die of something else. Even watchful-waiting opponents acknowledge that. Where urologists differ greatly is in determining for whom watchful waiting can safely be recommended.

The perplexing part of the prostate cancer equation stems from the fact that the cancer generally has an indolent nature—emphasis on "generally." You may have a generally placid pit bull, but that doesn't make you feel better if 1 percent of the time he snaps and bites the little girl next door. "A better question to ask than why 80 percent of it grows so slowly," says Dr. Chu of Roswell Park, "is why 20 percent of it grows so aggressively. We just don't know that yet."

So if there is resistance to the concept of simply monitoring cancer in the urological community, it's no surprise that the thought of not acting on it is frightening to the general populace. Always has been, probably always will be.

There is little mention of cancer in ancient history, possibly because it is to a large extent an age-related disease and people back then didn't live very long. According to Dr. Chu, who has researched the history, the word "cancer" was first used in the *Ebers Papyrus*, a significant Egyptian collection of medical texts from about 1500 BC. Others believe that the term owes its birth to Hippocrates, who used the Greek words *carcinos* or *karkinos* to describe "hard lumps" that were undoubtedly tumors. Hippocrates lived from about 460 BC to 377 BC. The Greek physician Herophilus, who lived from about 335 BC to 280 BC, first used the word "prostate" to describe that troublesome thing in front of the bladder.

(What we would've done without the ancient Greeks I do not know. But after that fast start, man, have they ever managed to screw things up.)

Cancer of the prostate was first identified in 1817 by a London physician named George Langstaff, but the disease goes back centuries. On October 26, 2011, the online *ScienceNOW* news site described the study of an Egyptian mummified 2,250 years ago and known as M1, who almost certainly had prostate cancer. M1, who is housed at the National Archaeological Museum in Lisbon, "struggled with a long, painful, progressive illness. A dull pain throbbed in his lower back, then spread to other parts of his body, making most movements a misery." That he had prostate cancer was determined by high-resolution scans, which showed, according to the magazine, "many small, round, dense tumors in M1's pelvis and lumbar spine, as well as in his upper arm and leg bones," the areas in which metastases most commonly occur.

Since I have previously compared the prostate to the breast in terms of public awareness, there also appears to be an evolutionary link between the two, that they "seem to have evolved on parallel tracks," as Dr. Walsh writes in *Surviving Prostate Cancer*. Countries with high breast cancer rates (including the United States, Great Britain, Australia) also have high prostate cancer rates, and countries with low breast cancer rates (most Asian nations) tend also to have low prostate cancer rates.

The thoughtful folks who communicated with me after I went public with my decision not to pursue intervention did not know of Egyptian mummies and Greek physicians. What they did know was that they had heard the word "cancer." Cancer is bad. Cancer kills. One of the cards I received was of a religious character and "hoped that God would find a way to heal me."

Half the population was telling me I wasn't sick, and the other was giving me last rites.

I can't emphasize this enough: I had no symptoms. One of the cards I received read "Hope you feel better," but there was nothing perceptibly wrong with me. When people who had read the newspaper column saw me at the gym, I could see them surreptitiously examining me for signs of deterioration and showing clear puzzlement when I didn't look any worse than I normally do.

The people I heard from about my active-surveillance decision were divided into two camps: One camp thought I was crazy but didn't say so, and the other thought I was crazy and did say so. My sister, Pam Scott, was in the former camp. Her husband, Chip, had been treated surgically for localized prostate cancer (his PSA number and Gleason score were similar to mine, and Dr. Lee had done his surgery) and she let me know, casually but emphatically, that he was doing fine except for some postsurgical "limitations."

Among those on the "You're nuts!" side was a local doctor who wrote me a heartfelt letter that read in part: "I have seen too many men die of prostate cancer. PLEASE PLEASE reconsider your decision not to get surgery."

That's pretty persuasive stuff when you're not 100 percent sure to begin with.

I consulted with Dr. Manley, who suggested I talk to a general oncologist. I bounced that idea off Keith, my urologist, and he had a better one:

Go to Johns Hopkins. See Ballentine Carter. He is The Man in active surveillance.

IT IS IMPOSSIBLE TO OVERSTATE the importance of Johns Hopkins University and its hospital to the study and treatment of prostate cancer. The first radical prostatectomy was performed there in 1904 by a surgeon named Hugh Hampton Young, and the procedure he used (removal of the whole gland and the seminal vesicles with the suturing together of the bladder and urethra) remained the model for four decades.

The highly regarded James Buchanan Brady Urological Institute on the hospital's Baltimore campus is not, however, named for a distinguished Hopkins urologist. Rather, it honors its benefactor, the famous, and famously overfed, "Diamond" Jim Brady, shady businessman, Broadway gadfly, and philanthropist. In 1912 Brady was successfully treated at Hopkins for various prostate problems—their existence perhaps not surprising considering his Herculean appetite—and in gratitude, he endowed the institute. A photo of Diamond Jim has a featured place in the staid Hopkins urology library, whose interior was designed, incidentally, by Margaret Walsh, wife of Dr. Patrick Walsh.

Dr. Walsh is probably the best known of Hopkins's dream team of urologists. He is credited not only with improving the "open" radical prostatectomy, which was once a downright barbaric procedure, but also with bringing prostate understanding to the masses with his teaching. Dr. Walsh still sees patients and does research (see Chapter 13 for more), and among his most distinguished colleagues is Dr. Carter, who is considered one of the leading practitioners of what the Hopkins team variously calls "expectant management with curative intent," "proactive monitoring," and "active surveillance."

When Hopkins adopted and refined the Swedish philosophy, they wanted nothing to do with the verb "waiting." They wanted to develop a proactive approach that involved PSA tests and rectal exams every six months, along with a yearly biopsy. We're Americans. We don't sit there and brood. We do stuff.

So I made an appointment with Dr. Carter, which took some doing—he is a busy man. His office requested not only my biopsy report, but also my biopsy slides.

The specifics of active surveillance are on the Hopkins Web site, as outlined by Dr. Carter and another urologist, Jonathan Epstein, MD. Their study has been going on for more than 15 years and has followed more than 900 men who, to quote the site, "are thought to have tumors that can be safely managed without immediate treatment."

Before the appointment, I would say that I perused the site. My wife digested it, and we formed the same opinion: Active surveillance seemed designed for men like me. As ol' Larry King might say, "Next to 'active surveillance' in the dictionary is a photo of Jack McCallum."

Dr. Carter met me late in the day. He had my records. He knew that my cancer was low level and had not escaped the prostate. He performed a digital rectal exam—expertly, I might add—and found nothing. Then he floored me with this pronouncement:

"You're 62. I would certainly not recommend active surveillance."

I was utterly confused. "Really? Why not?"

"Because of your age," he said. "And because you're in too good health. I know you weren't looking to be a patient down here, but, if you were, you would not be accepted into our program."

Dr. Carter said that the age of 65 is used, roughly, as a cutoff, but that a man's health is just as important. The healthier a man is, the more likely it is that he will die of prostate cancer because nothing else that is immediately evident will likely kill him. Therefore, it is advisable to kill the cancer. It makes a curious kind of sense, but you have to roll it around in your mind for a while.

I should've been happy, I suppose, since somebody had just told me that I was too young and too healthy for something, which hadn't happened in quite a while. But I walked out in a kind of daze. It was a long three-hour drive home, and my planned prostate solution was no solution at all.

CHAPTER 9

...In which the author visits an oncologist, changes strategies, communes with a robot, loses a walnut, and gains a catheter

MY WIFE AND I REREAD the Hopkins Web site page about the active-surveillance program, the address for which is in the Sources and Resources section at the back of this book. Here's what it says: "For older men, especially over age 65 years who meet criteria, active surveillance is one of the options that should be seriously considered." It also says the following: "Studies suggest that 30–50 percent of men over the age of 60 years diagnosed with prostate cancer today by PSA screening undergo a treatment that will not extend their life or improve its quality.... The key is to identify the men who for now can safely forego treatment."

That is where "life expectancy" comes in, which is, by definition, a free-floating estimate. It says, after all, "expectancy" not "certainty." The Hopkins people were not saying—could not know—that without surgical or radiological intervention I would die of prostate cancer because I was (at the time) 62 and in otherwise good health. Nor could they be sure that a cause other than "prostate cancer" would be on my death certificate. It was based on research, but it was basically a guess.

"Age is not the best criterion," says Dr. Walsh. "It's life span. There are 57-year-old men who aren't going to live 8 years, and there are 75-year-old men who are going to live 20 years."

When I was making this decision, I thought of myself as a 62-year-old who was more like a 52-year-old (albeit one with 72-year-old knees). At any rate, hearing that the country's top active-surveillance study would not accept me was a powerful disincentive to continue that protocol.

During my research, several active-surveillance advocates had also brought up the point that new tests, new medications, and improvements to the PSA test will almost certainly be coming along, as will genetic discoveries that will revolutionize prostate cancer detection. Hold off on intervention, the thinking was, and doctors would be able to more accurately assess whether my level of prostate cancer needed to be treated.

All that is true. But how far down the road are those new developments? Would I still be around? There is no way of knowing.

In retrospect, my decision to turn away from active surveillance began as soon as my appointment with Dr. Carter ended.

So now what? My literary agent, Scott Waxman, had been telling me that I should visit his father, a veteran oncologist at Mount Sinai Hospital in Manhattan. "Just see what he has to say," said Scott.

Samuel Waxman, MD, told me at the outset that he wasn't going to advise me on whether or not to get intervention. "That's not my job," he said. "I'm not a urologist. I'm not your doctor." He was familiar, of course, with both the ongoing controversy and the relatively slow advancement of prostate cancer. And over the course of a career spanning six decades, he had seen many patients die of prostate cancer. He understood the whole picture.

He examined me physically, giving me a pass on the DRE—"I suppose you've had enough of those," he said—and questioned my wife and me about our feelings on living with cancer, surgery, and possible post-intervention issues of incontinence and sexual dysfunction. He discussed his opinions about surgery and radiation. He touched all the bases. He was utterly complete and utterly professional without telling me what to do.

But one thing he said stuck with me more than anything else:

"The healthier you are going into surgery, the better you get through it. And you'll never be healthier or younger than you are right now."

True. I had never felt better. All right, that's a bunch of crap. I felt better when I was 30, when I could run six miles and play two hours of full-court basketball and report to work the next morning after tequila shots at midnight. But all in all, I felt good. So if surgery might be a necessity anyway—perhaps when I was 70 or 75—why not get it out of the way now?

I had also been thinking a lot about the active-surveillance regimen. I understood it, but had the feeling that I was unprepared to endure future biopsies, DREs, and constant PSA tests, all the while wondering if they were going to show something.

In the Sources and Resources section at the back of this book is the address for the Web site of an active-surveillance advocate, Michael Lasalandra. He is a medical journalist, so the info provided in his account of his cancer experience is clear, concise, and well written. It includes a full list of his PSA test results (from October 2006 through June 2012), which, after he started taking dutasteride (Avodart), went down from a high of 11.1 to a low of 3.3. But that isn't me. I didn't want to endlessly compile a list of my PSA readings. I didn't want to keep taking tests, wondering and worrying if the score was going to go up. If you're giving blood and visiting doctors and keeping logs, you are, in fact, obsessing, and, moreover, continuing to define yourself as Someone with Cancer.

I had finally told my sons (both of whom are in their 30s) that I had cancer, and they had given me their best "Are you kidding me?" reactions to the idea of active surveillance. The whole idea of waiting and watching never did catch hold with them, and it was beginning to lose favor with my wife, too. I had stopped talking about prostate cancer precisely because I didn't want to define myself by it. But one day I turned to my wife and said, "I thought I could forget I had cancer inside of me, but I can't. I think about it every time I urinate and every time we have sex."

She nodded. She had been thinking about it, too, and wondering why I had stopped talking about it. So as we strolled down Park Avenue after the appointment with Dr. Waxman, I turned to my wife and said, "I'm going to call Keith and tell him I'm having surgery."

She had been expecting it. "I'm glad," she said.

I told my family and friends of my decision to take action and they all seemed relieved, especially my sister.

"When you told me you weren't going to do anything," she said, "I thought you had lost your mind. But I've thought that before."

THE MORNING CALL
FEBRUARY 11, 2012

Being Convinced to Have Surgery
for Prostate Cancer

Some of you are at this moment muttering, "Wait a minute, we already heard about this guy's prostate. I'm trying to eat breakfast here."

I understand completely and won't feel slighted if you find something else to do. Tax season is upon us, after all, and it's not too early to start complaining about the Phillies' hitting.

But since I presented one side of the prostate case in a previous *Morning Call* column (Oct. 17, 2011), and since, for a while at least, I was the clearinghouse for Lehigh Valley prostate-cancer information, I feel obligated to reveal a change in my treatment decision.

Three months ago I was all but certain that I would embark upon a course called "active surveillance" or "watchful waiting." In prostate-cancer cases such as mine—low-level, relatively unaggressive, disease contained in the prostate—there is an argument for managing the disease without surgical or radiological intervention. You do this with more frequent PSA tests, digital-rectal exams and biopsies, counting on the fact that prostate cancer is slow growing.

I felt comfortable about that decision, and that's what I wrote in *The Morning Call* the first time. Almost immediately I received several phone calls and emails, most of a commiserating nature but others admonishing me for a wrong-headed decision. One was from a now-retired medical doctor. "You're making a big mistake," he said. "Get it taken care of surgically. Please."

(I appreciated all the messages, by the way, and they made me remember the number one benefit of writing for your local paper—an intimate connection with your readership. And I say that even though several readers wanted to string me up for a column about Penn State.)

Anyway, even with my tentative decision, I wasn't through researching. I made an appointment at The Johns

Hopkins Hospital with a doctor who specializes in active surveillance, thoroughly convinced that he would endorse my decision.

He did exactly the opposite.

"You're too young and too healthy," he said. "Go have the surgery." The Hopkins doctor was unequivocal and said he wouldn't have accepted me into his active-surveillance group if I were his patient.

It's been quite a while since anyone told me I was too young (62) and too healthy for anything, and my wife and I did have a couple of nice seafood meals in Baltimore. So the trip wasn't a total disaster.

But everything changed with the doctor's stark pronouncement. I continued to research the topic and it comes down to this: Like weekend football, prostate cancer is a game that comes with odds. They are free-floating and change as prostate research continues to trickle in, but you have to weigh those odds before making your treatment decision.

In cases such as mine, the odds are overwhelming that the cancer won't spread and/or kill me next year. Ten years from now? No one knows for sure, but my doctor at Penn tells me that, yes, he would bet that I would need intervention by then. Twenty years? The cancer would've almost certainly spread but maybe it still wouldn't have killed me. But maybe it would've. And since I don't have any other medical conditions at this time, the odds on the big board say that prostate cancer would ultimately be my cause of death.

Further, a Mount Sinai oncologist I saw—this thing started to take on the characteristics of a United Nations fact-finding mission—would not advise me one way or the other but did make this point: The healthier you go into surgery, the better your odds of coming out of it OK. Right now I have no complicating issues except a bum left knee and a tendency to hit my mid-irons flat.

So, I will be having surgery. I could write an entire column on why I went for robotic instead of traditional and why I chose surgery over radiation, but a little morning disease conversation goes a long way. My procedure is set for Feb. 20, and my hope is that it will be so uneventful that a third column will be unnecessary. Hey, that might be your hope, too.

Jim Boeheim, who has been the basketball coach at Syracuse University since Moses led the Israelites across the desert, told me that he was entirely satisfied with the traditional method of prostate removal—the "open" procedure. His had been performed by one of the reigning kings of prostate cancer, Dr. William Catalona, who is adamant about the open procedure being better than its robotic alternative. I discussed it with Dr. Catalona in his Chicago office after my surgery, and he subsequently sent me his PowerPoint presentation that extols the virtues of the open surgery.

The final slide carries this notation: "The Most Important Factor." The image shows one surgeon bent over a console and the other standing over a patient. The message is clear. "I always tell my patients that 'feel' is the most important thing," said Dr. Catalona. "You can be blind and be a great musician and you can be deaf and be a great writer, but if you're a surgeon, you're giving up something when you surrender sense of touch."

Dr. Catalona also said the virtues of robotic surgery have been oversold, that the da Vinci people and overly aggressive hospital marketers have presented the robot as a panacea, exaggerating, both expressly and obliquely, its benefits. I have no doubt that is true. There is the suggestion that the robot has been imbued with magical curative powers when, in fact, most evenhanded robotic surgeons will tell you that, in terms of surgical safety and postoperative recovery of urinary and sexual function, there are few differences between the open and robotic methods—if they are done by skilled and experienced people.

"People like Dr. Catalona and Dr. Walsh have done so many open procedures that their performance and outcomes are consistent," says Dr. Lee. "Their patients do really, really well because of their skill as an open surgeon."

Dr. Catalona trained under Dr. Walsh, who perfected the nerve-sparing open technique in the early 1980s, paving the way for tens of thousands of men to have their prostates removed without permanent loss of potency or urinary control. Dr. Walsh, now 75, stopped operating in 2011—"Always leave when you're at the top of your game," he told me, which is roughly what legendary running back Jim Brown said after he retired despite still being near his prime—and made it clear that, as he sees it, no robot is (or ever could be) as good as he was.

"My patients went home either the next morning or the following morning, they got their catheter out at nine days, they had a three-inch incision, they were taking no pain medication, and they were continent," says Dr. Walsh. "The results were exactly the same as with the robotic."

Surgeons tend not to be the shrinking violets of the world, but I have no doubt that Dr. Walsh speaks the truth. Mention "Walsh" at a urological symposium and watch for widespread genuflection to break out. But people like Dr. Walsh and Dr. Catalona cannot be present at every procedure, and, as Dr. Walsh concedes, open surgery is more difficult to perform. This is because the larger incision it requires causes greater blood loss than the smaller ones made for laparoscopic robotic surgery, and blood in the surgical field can obscure the anatomy and make maneuvering less controllable—increasing the risk to the patient. "There is no doubt that the advantage of the robotic is that all this bleeding is reduced," says Dr. Walsh, "and you can see better because there is less blood loss." In OR terms, robotic surgeons generally look at a "bloodless field," and that translates into generally no need for blood transfusions to replace what's lost.

Also, post-op recovery is undoubtedly quicker for robotic patients than it is for open patients. "If you see patients who just had robotic and patients who just had open," says the University of Rochester's Dr. Edward Messing, who is himself an open surgeon, "you don't have to be a genius to see which is which. Sure, the hospital stay is only a day less with the robotic, but that's because we're pretty brutal in kicking patients out of the hospital."

The bottom line is: Dr. Walsh, who perfected the open procedure, has not dug a moat to drown the advancing brigade of robotic surgeons. As director of the Brady Urological Institute for 30 years, he witnessed the coming of the robot a decade ago and didn't stand in the way. There are open surgeons and robotic surgeons on the Hopkins staff, and they don't have daily food fights in the lunchroom. Dr. Lee is among the thousands who have visited Hopkins to observe surgical techniques.

There is ongoing financial controversy about the robot—what isn't there controversy about in the prostate cancer world?—and it's safe to assume that insurers have spent many hours comparing the costs of both approaches. Some studies have already concluded that the robot costs more. Dr. Lee says that is not the case. "Both the per-case cost and the OR cost are more expensive with the robot," he says. "But the hospital stay is shorter. We did a cost analysis and the procedures turned out to be pretty equal because the robot saved money on [length of] stay and blood transfusion."

Looking ahead, one does wonder if the USPSTF recommendation against PSA testing will bring down the number of cancer diagnoses, thereby bringing down the number of surgical interventions—and the likelihood of a hospital spending something around $2 million on a robot.

On the other hand, the future surgeons being taught in medical school right now are increasingly embracing the robot. "Once they get their hands on it, it's hard to get them off," says Dr. Lee. "Look, the open procedure, when it's not done by skilled guys, can be messy."

But all that was background noise as far as my decision making went. Let's be honest: Most people take the Ayn Rand route on medical decisions—self-interest above all. What's good for me, not the health care world as a whole, is what I'm going to do. I wasn't about to calculate the costs of my choice to the health care system. With the insurance plan I have, I was going to be out-of-pocket for a couple thousand dollars anyway.

So from the beginning I knew I would choose the robotic method. Keith was an advocate of it even though he didn't do it himself. He had utter faith in Dr. Lee, whom I studied up on and learned that he had performed his 3,000-plus procedures without a fatality. I wanted limited blood loss and a quick recovery. I have nothing against robots. I loved Woody Allen's *Sleeper*.

I made an appointment with Dr. Lee's office. It was January 12, 2012, by this time. So here is my prostate cancer time line:

- **Rising PSA detected in July 2011**
- **Biopsy on September 7**
- **Fairly firm intention to choose active surveillance until November 2, the date of my appointment with Dr. Carter at Johns Hopkins**
- **Choice switched to surgery after my appointment with Dr. Waxman on November 29**
- **Pre-op appointment with Dr. Lee's office on January 12**
- **Surgery set for February 20, 2012**

A seven-month arc in all.

During that January appointment, one of Dr. Lee's staff members went over the preliminaries. Arrive at the hospital in the morning.

Procedure would take between two and three hours. An hour or so in recovery. Wake up in my hospital room and stay only one night as long as there are no complications. Leave with a catheter and a supply of pain medication, etc. She also gave me an instruction sheet detailing how to do Kegel exercises, the pelvic squeezing movements that are designed to improve post-op continence.

"I have every reason to believe you'll come through this fine," Dr. Lee said when he arrived for a brief conference.

Easy for him to say. But his confidence was comforting.

ONE HAS TO BE CAREFUL not to enter the I'm Special Because I Have Cancer Club. I didn't have symptoms. My life was not disrupted. There was nothing heroic or tragic about my having cancer. My story was different from that of a five-year-old battling brain cancer who heads off to kindergarten bald, a woman going to bed with her partner for the first time after a mastectomy, a man with a colostomy bag standing up and checking his trousers before stepping to the podium to make a speech.

My story was different from that of my friend Dale Briggs, who lived with pancreatic cancer for two years, never complaining, never talking about it, kayaking, hiking, and enjoying life as if nothing was the matter. Pancreatic cancer continues to defy researchers because, in the words of cancer researcher Dr. Chu, "There are no early pancreatic patients." The disease arrives stealthily, presents with relatively unremarkable symptoms ("I have a little backache"), and kills quickly and efficiently.

So there was no reason to obsess about the operation, and most people around me forgot I had a procedure scheduled. But why not play the cancer card when it can be helpful, right? At the time, I was finishing up a book on the 1992 Olympic Dream Team and still had not secured an interview with one key player—Boston Celtics legend Larry

Bird, then the president of the NBA's Indiana Pacers. He had rebuffed my attempts on several occasions, and 10 days before my operation I made one last call to his assistant, Susy Fischer.

"Tell Larry I'm having cancer surgery," I said, "and if I die on the table my last thought will be that he blew me off."

I said it in a semijocular manner but with enough seriousness to (hopefully) push the guilt button. Bird called me back. I made an appointment, flew to Indianapolis two days later, and did the interview. With the tape recorder off, Bird and I spent a few minutes discussing the prostate, erections, peeing, and the general horrors of two men growing old.

THERE ARE FEW THINGS MORE DEPRESSING than the predawn slog to the hospital for surgery. The sleepy-eyed receptionist taking your information like you're the least interesting person on earth. The low, drowsy hum of hospital machinery coming to life. The strange isolation of the prep room with that open-in-the-back robe whose fabric has been graced by a thousand foreign buttocks. The wary glances of other patients waiting to be cut open, all of us wondering, *Are you in worse shape than I am?* And worst of all, the donning of those pressure stockings, designed to prevent blood clots, that make me think of Richard Nixon and his soul-killing phlebitis.

All in all, you feel like this just might be the Last Roundup.

An orderly came to get me. "I see you're having surgery with Dr. Lee," he told me. "The man has magic hands."

I didn't know whether that was part of the Penn Presbyterian rap, but I appreciated it.

"You'll have to leave him here," he said to my wife. There were traces of wetness in the corners of her eyes.

"Next time you see me I'll have a catheter in me," I said.

"Yes, but you won't have any cancer in you," she said, her lips brushing mine.

I don't want to make this overly dramatic because I wasn't going in for brain surgery or anything like that. But a line from *The Virgin Suicides* came to mind, the part where the author, Jeffrey Eugenides, paraphrased T. S. Eliot: "She was the still point in a turning world." So I wanted to make Donna the last thing I saw if she was, for whatever reason, the last thing I saw.

The anesthesiologist performed his magic and soon I was in dreamland, that strange interruption of the time–space continuum. You somehow hope that you'll come back a little younger or a little smarter, or at the very least find that something significant happened, movement on the Palestinian situation or the announcement that *Breaking Bad* had been renewed for nine seasons.

Nothing like that happened, though, and by 11:00 a.m. I was awake in my room, Donna seated on a chair beside my bed reading a magazine. I was feeling sore in the abdominal area as a hideous cocktail of blood, urine, and God knows what else drip-drip-dripped into a bag from the goddamn catheter that now defined my existence. I had gas pains. I wasn't hungry at all, which is a good indication that something had happened.

But I was alive and didn't feel that bad, all things considered.

Everybody assured me that the operation had gone smoothly, and one of the nurses who checked my stitches said, "Dr. Lee, right? I'd recognize his work anywhere." Did they hand out cue cards at employee indoctrination? Or was the guy just that good?

The day passed slowly. I got out of bed a half-dozen times, walking better and better but with some abdominal pain and utterly conscious of my catheter, afraid it would suddenly slip out and start spraying urine like an anarchic garden hose. But the night passed without incident. Most of the rooms at Penn Presbyterian are private, and that is a major blessing. During hospital stays, I would hand over my life savings for privacy.

The next morning Dr. Lee came in and announced that everything was fine. "Your prostate was normal-sized and the procedure only took 90 minutes," he said. "That is good. I spared as many nerves as I could. You should have a good outcome. You're scheduled to come back and see me in a week."

"Thanks, Doc," I said. "But, look, why don't we save ourselves some time. Yank this catheter out right now and we'll call it a day."

He laughed. He had probably heard that one before.

"You need it," he said. "It takes time for everything to repair down there. But I'll see you soon."

"You want to take a look at the stitches before you leave?" I asked.

"No need to," he said.

Okay, that was badass. The man was so confident he didn't even have to look at his work. Patients tend to think of their procedures as special and precious things, models to be studied by doctors and nurses. They're not. Dr. Lee was happy that things had gone well, obviously, but here's what my post-op day was for him: Tuesday.

Before my wife and I left, a nurse gave us detailed instructions about the Foley catheter. The patient will usually refer to it simply as a "catheter" or "that f—ing thing strapped to my leg," but hospital folks respectfully include the adjective "Foley" and sometimes just call it a "Foley." I wonder if its inventor, Frederic Foley, a Boston surgeon in the 1930s, was proud of it, or, more to the point, if his family was: "Yeah, my dad came up with the thingie that goes into men's penises so they can carry around their own urine." All in all, not conversation for the high school cafeteria.

(An early flexible catheter, by the way, was developed by Ben Franklin—what didn't that guy stick his nose in?—who used it to ease his brother's pain from kidney stones and also to play childish pranks on serious-minded Alexander Hamilton during the Constitutional Convention. Okay, I made one of those up.)

I'm not a systems guy. I don't like straps, buckles, and tubes—particularly when they're going into my penis, through my urethra, and into my bladder—and asked my wife to please pay close attention to the catheter instructions.

You leave the hospital with the big bag, the one you carry like an obscene oversized purse, as if fulfilling some medieval punishment imposed by the church. The little bag is the one you wear in public. It straps easily to the side of your knee. The nurse told me that showering, blessedly, would not be a problem as long as I didn't scrub at the incision sites. You simply disconnect the tube from the bag and clip it off, and you don't even need to use the clip if you don't mind urine running down the drain. I did not, though my wife might've had another opinion. It was freedom. It also sounds like a plot device for an episode of *Curb Your Enthusiasm*.

Needless to say, the catheter consumes your every thought. You're kind of amazed, first of all, at the thickness of the thing. Shouldn't it be thinner if it's going to fit in there? Jeff Jarvis, the writer, refers to the act of removing a catheter as a "hosectomy."

When you wear the big bag, you have more of a pulling sensation because, obviously, there is considerable weight on the other end from both the bag itself and the urine it's holding. You don't have that when you wear the small bag, but then you worry about potential spillover. That did happen to me once. Fortunately, I was in my bedroom, not in the public library.

Catheterized, you exist in a kind of purgatory, between epochs— BC (Before Catheter) and AD (After Displacement). When you're awake, you have the constant fear that it's coming out, and when you're asleep you dream that you're driving through West Virginia, it slips out, you pull over, and a gas station attendant who resembles the banjo kid in *Deliverance* has to reinsert it.

On my third day with the catheter, I got a call from a friend, Mike Caruso, a former three-time NCAA wrestling champion, who one year earlier had undergone a robotic prostatectomy with Dr. Lee.

"You doing okay?" he asked.

"Yeah, but this catheter sucks," I said. "It pulls at you and it seems like all I do is change the bag. Or my wife does. I gotta tell you, it's no picnic around here."

"But you get it out soon," he said. "And that feeling? I can tell you it's better than winning Nationals."

CHAPTER 10

...In which the author celebrates catheter removal, gets his postsurgical pathology report, and skulks around in search of pads

THE PERIOD IMMEDIATELY FOLLOWING SURGERY feels like a regression in time. You become a child, every minor accomplishment a triumph, every bodily-function milestone a joyful celebration.

"Oh, that's a good burp. Are you starting to feel better?"

"Oh, you just passed gas. *Wonderful!*"

The first post-op bowel movement is the most significant milestone. They frequently forget to tell you at the hospital that painful constipation can be a consequence of the terrible triad of anesthesia, pain medication, and mostly being flat on your back, but I am a post-op veteran and was determined it was not going to happen. So in the days immediately following my surgery I stayed away from protein and all but starved myself on a diet of soup, juice, and water. You don't know what a sacrifice that is unless you've seen me perform a graceful pas de deux with a plate of sausage. I took short walks constantly, wearing baggy sweatpants and waving jauntily to my neighbors with one hand while using the other to check that my catheter was still engaged.

With the help of stool softeners—do not abuse them, but for God's sake don't ignore them—I had the bowel issue worked out four days after surgery. As I congratulated myself, I noticed I was bleeding at the tip of the catheter. I called Keith, my urologist. Here's what his life is like: He picked up, having just come out of the operating room for an emergency procedure. It was nine o'clock on a Friday night.

"A little bleeding is natural," Keith said. "It comes from straining. Obviously if it continues, give me a call. But you'll be fine."

It stopped. And to be honest I didn't have a major catheter issue. I kept moving constantly; one night between 1:00 and 2:00 a.m., I trekked a path around the bottom floor of the house 137 times. I counted. It passed the time. So did *Law and Order* reruns, which I began to imagine were an homage to Jerry Orbach—who played Detective Lennie Briscoe—a prostate cancer fatality.

No matter how you pass the time, you never forget that the catheter is in. It confirms, by its very existence and positioning, one of the male's worst fears—that his penis is shrinking. You are supposed to check the catheter area from time to time to see if it's black and blue, which means you're constantly looking down, which means you see the catheter seemingly pushing your penis farther and farther into your body.

Plus, there's this: Your member might, in fact, actually *be* shrinking. A University of Miami study found that in nearly 20 percent of prostatectomy patients, penile length decreased by at least 15 percent. You know how you're supposed to "do the math"? I don't want to do the math on that. Dr. Lee theorizes that shrinkage could happen over time because of poor circulation during that period when men are not having erections. "The oxygen content gets so low it's scary," he says, "and if that state continues for a year or 15 months, that tissue stays firm, not spongy. So when a guy has an erection it stays more contracted."

I've noticed a burgeoning cottage industry in reporting on the possibility of reduced penis size and there is still much research to be done (if anyone really wants to take it on). A link to one theory about it is listed in the Sources and Resources section at the back of the book. But the message from urologists seems to be a positive one: Use it or lose it. My wife tells me that something similar is conveyed to menopausal women by their gynecologists. How nice it is when sexual missives actually intersect in the marital ether.

During a day of Googling—one tends to spend a lot of catheter time Googling—I came across a Web site on which men and women talked about enjoying sexual activity while their Foley catheters were in. Perhaps I was getting conservative in my old age, but that didn't spark even the slightest bit of curiosity.

The real sexual questions were going to emerge after the catheter did.

WHICH IT DID EASILY AND WITH A QUIET SNAP that was one of the most blissful sounds I ever heard. The balloon at the bladder end of the tube is deflated before extraction and there's nothing to it. Kelly Monahan—Dr. Lee's PA, whom you remember from Leonard Collier's operation—said it wouldn't hurt, and it didn't. It had been in for eight days. It felt like eight years, but now it was over.

"Tell me something, Kelly, and I mean this sincerely," I said. "What's a nice girl like you doing in a place like this?"

She laughed. So did my wife, who was along for the appointment. Kelly said she enjoyed the whole urology package—assisting Dr. Lee, who appreciates her input, the team approach, the buzz of the OR, being able to prescribe medication, giving men and their partners positive news, which she says is what she mostly does after Dr. Lee's robotic prostatectomies.

She said she had some for me, in fact.

"I have your post-op pathology report," she said. "Let's see . . . your prostate weighed 39.7 grams [about 1.4 ounces]. That's about normal. The pathologists biopsied the gland and your Gleason was 3 + 4. That's a little change, just a little worse, from the 3 + 3 pre-op. You had clear margins, but the cancer had advanced near the capsule.

"When your prostate came out it was in one big piece with the seminal vesicles attached. Pathology covers the whole thing with ink, which then represents the margins. We want the margins to be clean. Cancer sometimes invades the seminal vesicles from the prostate and can spread outside of one or both. That produces a positive margin. But yours were negative. You are cancer-free."

I don't care how low your level of cancer was, how confident you were going in, or how much somebody said that you didn't need surgery—hearing the words "cancer-free" will make your day. And the fact that my cancer was one Gleason point more serious, as well as a little closer to the capsule, i.e., the outer edge of the gland, made me feel better about having gotten it out.

Kelly explained—though we'd already known—that any future orgasms would be dry since the semen-manufacturing vesicles had been hauled out with the prostate. She suggested waiting two to three weeks for sexual activity. "We encourage it after that," she added, "because it will help the healing." Dr. Marvin Gaye advocated a similar "Sexual Healing" treatment, and by most accounts took his own advice.

"So it was a good report," continued Kelly, "and I'm glad you had your prostate removed. So is Dr. Lee. You should feel the same way."

"I do," I said. And I did.

The rest of the discussion centered on pads, so much talk about pads that I could've been at a training session for Kotex salesmen. "Leakage can be a real problem," she said. "Some men tell me they use one pad every other day, others have told me they go through six or seven a day. Did you do your Kegel exercises before surgery?"

I could've said that I was the Kegel King, but I told the truth.

"I'd give myself a C in that department," I said.

I don't have a reason for not having been better at it. I could tell Kelly wanted to give me a lecture, but, hey, I just spent eight days in Catheter Incarceration.

Then she released me with this chilling admonition: "We want you to urinate as soon as possible. If you can't, if you have urinary retention, you should go to the emergency room immediately. About 2 percent of men have to be recatheterized."

"Excuse me?" I said. "Recatheterized? When you're awake?"

"Some men are unable to urinate," she said. "There's a blockage. It probably won't happen. You should be fine. But don't delay doing something about it if it does."

My wife and I thanked Kelly and immediately adjourned to the hospital cafeteria, where I drank enough water to quench the thirst of the entire Kentucky Derby starting field. You're familiar with the expression "piss like a racehorse"? That was my intention.

But not my outcome. I stood over the hopper for a minute or two as thoughts of recatheterization and images of the *Deliverance* kid wearing a hospital orderly's uniform came into my head until . . . something appeared to be happening. I couldn't feel much of anything—the nerves still were not back—but I was urinating, slowly and anything but surely, but doing it for the first time in eight days on my own. Not much came out. But whatever came out felt wonderful, if only as a psychic release.

I placed a phone call to Mike Caruso when I got home. "Congratulate me, Mike," I said. "I just won Nationals."

As a teen, your heart beat like a tom-tom when you slipped that copy of *Playboy* in between the daily newspaper and the sports magazine, and when you tried to hide that package of condoms amid an unholy assemblage of gum and candy bars. So one of the joys of getting old is that you're not generally embarrassed during shopping.

Unless you're a post-prostatectomy victim on your first excursion for pads.

"Can't you just buy them for me?" I said to my wife.

"I don't know what's right," she said, no doubt flashing a secret smile that meant *You never shopped for* my *pads.*

Pads, pads, pads, pads, pads, pads, pads. Every prostate questionnaire I filled out before and after surgery included questions about urination—Drippage? All-out leakage? Feelings of not being finished? How soaked are your pads? Minimally soaked? Utterly soaked? Desperately, existentially, Nietzsche-level soaked?

I had gotten dire warnings about control issues. One man called my house and admonished my wife, "Be sure to get those waterproof protective pads that go between the bottom sheet and the mattress pad. You're going to need them." He sounded like a meteorologist describing a particularly powerful and unpredictable monsoon heading for shore.

From the beginning, though, I felt fairly confident that I would be continent. But I couldn't be sure, so after getting my catheter removed my wife and I headed to the store.

My sons had named their high school band Aisle Nine after a song they wrote about that overlooked lane in the market where all the strange products were kept—Spam, off-brand candy, particularly revolting species of canned fish. The pads are near that area of Wegmans, in a far corner under a sign identifying the entire section as INTIMATE CARE and specifically INCONTINENCE. It was the section where you didn't want to meet any of your friends who might be passing by on the way to the nearby PAIN RELIEF section:

Hey, Jack. Listen, I heard about your cancer. You doing okay?

Sure, Bob. Doing great. I'm looking for avocados. Gonna make some kickass guacamole.

Right. But they'd probably be in produce, all the way at the other end of the store. You're in the incontinence section.

Oh, hell, didn't even notice. Thanks.

My wife and I perused the sad offerings. The products had names designed to inspire confidence. Depend. Poise. Prevail. Certainty. The euphemistic coyness made sense, I suppose, being much better than a product packaged as I Might Be Peeing Right Now but You Wouldn't Know It. We finally settled on a box of pads, a box of smaller guards, and the climax to this dispiriting trifecta—incontinence briefs, an oversized something that looked like they were made for a laugh line in an Austin Powers movie.

"These are kind of like what Oliver wears," she said, speaking of our 2-year-old grandson, who was going through potty training at the time.

"I'm announcing right now that those will never come out of the box," I said. "If it comes to the point where I have to wear them, I will stay inside. I will become Howard Hughes."

My wife didn't have a lot of sympathy. "Imagine being a 12-year-old girl and hearing your mother explain, 'Pin these to your underwear, and by the way you'll be bleeding for the next 40 years.' So stop complaining."

So I stopped complaining.

Each morning for the first couple of weeks after the catheter removal I dutifully put on the big pad and felt like I was walking around with a banana between my legs. I was in sweatpants most of the time. I took the pad off at night and threw it away and except for minor exceptions the pads were always dry. Then I moved to the smaller pad, and after a few days I didn't wear anything.

I got lucky. I am not taking credit for having urinary control after surgery, because I had cheated on my Kegel exercises. I give credit for my success to Dr. Lee and to the fact that I hadn't been incontinent before surgery.

We eventually donated all the pads and guards to a prostate support group, except for a single pair of the Austin Powers briefs. You never know when you might need something for Halloween.

CHAPTER 11

... In which the author rejects Levitra, finds Cialis, puts his oars into different sexual waters, and finds satisfaction, if not fireworks

IN MY CATHETER-REMOVAL DEBRIEFING, Kelly had not said much about a timetable for the return of sexual function because there was not much to say. It's a mystery. The nerves responsible for erections are not in the prostate, as was once believed. Rather, they are located on each side of the prostate. They run along the urethra and come out into the pelvic area and the penis. If both nerves are damaged or removed during treatment, a man probably won't be able to have an erection without the aid of medication or some kind of device. Spare one set of nerves or both and a man has a decent shot of regaining good sexual function, depending, of course, on his age and potency going in.

Surgeons will give you a fair assessment for the return of function, but "fair" is about as far as anyone will go. No surgeon, no matter how confident, is going to march in and proclaim: "Nerve sparing was complete. Tell your partner to start microwaving the lotion. You're about to get busy again, playa!"

In my case, Dr. Lee shaded toward optimism about both continence and erectile function. "A human being's peripheral nerves are covered by a strong, fibrous layer that protects them from injury," says Dr. Lee. "When you hit your funny bone it hurts, but your nerves don't die. Well, the nerves that control unconscious things like bladder and erection function don't have that same kind of covering. So any kind of stretch, pull, or tearing makes them a lot more susceptible." Nevertheless, he still envisioned a positive outcome for me.

As part of the post-op reboot of the reproductive system, Dr. Lee's urology group prescribes daily erectile dysfunction medication. It's not designated for immediate sexual activity, but, rather, for aiding in the long-term return of blood flow. Their prescription for me called for a 20-milligram (mg) dose of vardenafil (Levitra).

I didn't have too much experience with ED medication except for a few liaisons with sildenafil (Viagra). It worked okay, but gave me severe nasal congestion.

"I'm not going to do this anymore," I told my wife.

"That's fine," said Donna, a retired teacher. "You sound like one of my sniffling second-graders in January."

Mostly I knew ED medication from its inane advertising campaigns. Couples fox-trotting in the kitchen. Couples on a porch swing giving each other touches freighted with meaning. Couples lounging al fresco in . . . different bathtubs? How is that supposed to work exactly? Mutual telepathic masturbation? In one Cialis (tadalafil) spot, the bathtubs are replaced by inner tubes, which would make mutual telepathic masturbation even more difficult, water being a poor frictional conductor.

When those commercials first came out, several politicians were offended—or pretended to be—by the suggestiveness of the ads. The FDA banned a couple of the ED ads, which they labeled "misleading" because they failed to disclose major side effects.

And if you think there can't be major side effects, you weren't with me on the night of March 1, 2012, after I took my first 20 mg dose of Levitra. Congestion so bad I had trouble breathing. Parched throat. Severe headache bordering on a migraine. Hot flashes—go ahead and laugh, women—so intense that I felt like I was being incinerated. It was much, much worse than any of the eight nights I had experienced with the catheter.

I called Kelly. She had never heard of a reaction that severe, but she did note that men react differently to similar dosages of similar drugs. No one knows why. It's just another of life's delicious mysteries. She switched me to a 5 mg dosage of Cialis. Since then it's been fine, though I continue to favor shower stalls over bathtubs.

ON A DARK LATE-WINTER AFTERNOON, candles and incense burning, I made torrid love to my wife.

"You're incredible," she said, her head resting on my strong left shoulder. "It's like nothing even happened to you. It's like you're 30 years old again. It's like you're . . . you're . . . Superman."

Then we fell asleep in each other's arms, waking only to start over again and . . .

Okay, I made that up.

Let me say that this next part is not easy for my wife or me. Especially her. Donna is an intensely private person, and, though I am less so, I do not routinely discuss our sex life. Sex is all you talk about when you're 20 and something you barely mention when you're 60. I didn't say you didn't do it; you just don't talk about it. But post-prostatectomy sexual reports have to be part of this account, so I'm going all in.

So to speak.

The first post-op sexual encounter, which happened about three weeks after the catheter was removed, had a lab-experiment feel to it. I didn't expect anyone's earth to move, least of all the section on which my wife was reclining, and it didn't. I felt aroused like always—even after 40 years I find my wife very attractive very quickly—but I couldn't get a full erection. And I am used to achieving full erections quickly. I would put my erection at 60 percent, but perhaps that's influenced by the normal male exaggeration about anything to do with sex, so let's put it at 40 percent.

Being with my wife was certainly a pleasant way to pass the time, far superior to beating a path around the downstairs perimeter 137 times. We stopped and talked and started again and talked some more, much more talking than usual. Then we started again and, suddenly—

In their landmark sex study, Masters and Johnson coined the phrase "ejaculatory inevitability" to describe the moment during stimulation when a man feels orgasm is inevitable. They further concluded that men reach orgasm after two or fewer minutes of masturbation, or, as I prefer to call it, self-inflicted orgasm (SIO). I buy the inevitability fact—at least I've always found it to be the case—but disbelieve the SIO statistic. Two or fewer minutes seems a little quick, doesn't it? Particularly if you're in a bathtub.

I would guess that most post-prostatectomy patients aren't confident about ejaculatory inevitability, or, in its amended form, dry-ejaculatory inevitability. A prostatectomy forces one to think about the whole complicated process of orgasm, a topic that, like sausage making, lessens in appeal when overanalyzed. The production of an orgasm necessitates a cooperative assembly line that involves the testicles, the epididymis (a tube that connects the efferent ducts at the rear of each testicle to its vas deferens), the vas deferens, the urethra, the penis, and, most of all, the brain.

The prostate is not needed for orgasm, but with all the bodily changes and your confidence level down, you don't know if it's going to happen and, if it does, whether you'll recognize it. Perhaps it will pass by so fast that it will be vaguely familiar yet ultimately unidentifiable, like a particularly exotic make of foreign car whooshing by on the highway. But, suddenly—

It happened. I had an orgasm. It came (excuse verb choice) unexpectedly and with a limited erection. Consequently, it didn't feel complete. But the feeling was intense, possibly because those muscles had not been used for a while. It might've been akin to the first time I ejaculated, though I don't remember that. Afterward, my penis felt tingly, as if somebody had rapped it with one of those small hammers used to test reflexes.

My first response was that I could not believe there was no ejaculate. I looked for it. None. Completely dry. There are reports of men having full ejaculate after a prostatectomy, but, then again, there are reports of Virgin Mary sightings in chicken cacciatore. (Actually, a small amount of ejaculate fluid can be produced in the prostate's neighboring Cowper's glands, but even that is fairly rare.)

"What did it feel like?" Donna asked.

"I guess I would say its suddenness made it intense," I answered. "But it felt kind of... incomplete."

I thought about it for a while. "I think I have a new name for it," I said. "The no-gasm."

"You're not being fair," Donna said. "Men who can't have an orgasm of any kind have no-gasms. This was at least a gasm of some kind."

Point taken. No-gasm is officially stricken from my post-prostatectomy vocabulary.

How about half-gasm? Better yet—faux-gasm.

From a performance standpoint, the experience should not be in my top 100 sexual memories. But it is. It was a good moment. Life will go on. It will be different. But it will go on.

And as we lay there, Donna couldn't resist this:

"How do I know," she began, framing a question that has no doubt been asked by a thousand partners of prostatectomy graduates, "that you weren't faking it?"

CHAPTER 12

...In which the author learns a few things he should've paid more attention to before surgery

ABOUT EIGHT WEEKS AFTER SURGERY, I got the contract to do this book. I had already begun taking notes, having been convinced by the response to my newspaper columns that there was much interest in, and confusion about, this subject. So I began talking in earnest to doctors and regular folks about prostate cancer.

My first surprise was the concern about biopsies, primarily the possibility of contracting infection, most commonly called urosepsis. I have nothing but overall praise for the information my doctors gave me throughout this process, but I will say that the potential perils of the biopsy were undersold—in fact, not sold at all. Perhaps that is my fault since I didn't do any research on it. My main concern was to be blissfully unaware of the harpooning procedure, wake up, and go on my way.

Or perhaps doctors don't say much about it because the risk of infection seems so self-evident. After all, the procedure involves inserting a needle that passes through the rectum en route to the prostate. That is problematic territory, and to not anticipate trouble would be like Custer expecting a cakewalk as he led the Seventh Cavalry through Montana.

The use of smaller needles has made the procedure better—"It used to be a horrendous undertaking," says Dr. Pablo Torre, the Department of Veterans Affairs urologist—but "less horrendous" doesn't necessarily translate into "less dangerous." And "dangerous" is precisely the word used by my urologist, who is not given to scary proclamations for the hell of it.

"In the last two years we've had two 50-year-old men die from their prostate biopsies," says Dr. Keith Van Arsdalen. "And it's not like we're doing something wrong. I suspect our record is pretty good, in fact. It's just that a biopsy can be a dangerous procedure."

Dr. Jerry Blaivas, the New York City urologist, says that at least 1 percent and possibly as many as 4 percent of men who have prostate biopsies get serious infections. "So if you're a 62-year-old man and you keep getting biopsies," says Dr. Blaivas, "eventually you're going to get a life-threatening infection."

Dr. Lee says he feels comfortable saying that the accurate figure is closer to 1 percent. "But that is still significant," says Dr. Lee, "because the guys who get it are really sick. I have never lost a patient going through prostate cancer surgery, but I had a patient die going through a prostate biopsy. And the infections can be antibiotic resistant. So if the first two antibiotics don't work, a guy keeps getting sicker and sicker, and by the time they find the right one he has one foot in the grave.

"What we should remember, though, is that antibiotic-resistant organisms are not exclusively a problem of prostate biopsies. They are a problem that affects all areas of medicine."

Numerous studies have confirmed the existence of high infection rates and at least one postulated that after three biopsies a man could become impotent. "It is important for urologists to determine if a biopsy is appropriate for an individual patient," says Dr. Ballentine Carter regarding a Johns Hopkins study, "and also if the patient is at increased risk for a biopsy-related complication."

One of Dr. Carter's distinguished colleagues isn't quite so pessimistic. "A more recent study [from the University of California at San Francisco] showed that that wasn't the case," says Dr. Walsh. "And I absolutely don't consider fear of biopsy a reasonable deterrent to intervention, if intervention is needed."

But every man has to make that decision on his own. Would the possibility, be it 1, 2, 3, or 4 percent, of a serious infection make you reluctant to get a biopsy? I can only answer for myself: It would not. That's just how I am. I would have taken that chance even if I had known about the infection potential. Somebody else might not.

"I do not buy biopsy danger as a deterrent to getting a PSA test, as the USPSTF does," says Dr. Lee. "But the biopsy technology could definitely get better, and the profession knows it. There's some research going on in Israel right now in the form of a new antibiotic-impregnated needle. And in those tests the infection rate has gone down to almost zero."

As a further horror, there is in the prostate playbook something called "saturation biopsy." You've heard of saturation bombing? This is metaphorically the same thing, but with your prostate as the target. Between 30 and 80 cores are taken, usually in men who seem to be at high risk for prostate cancer yet have had negative results on their previous biopsies. I'd talk that one over with my physician very, very carefully.

ANOTHER THING I STARTED TO HEAR A LOT ABOUT—after the fact— was Urorad facilities. The word sounds like something that might come from the mouth of a 17-year-old ("Dude, I just heard Toy, and they are totally Euro-rad"), but it refers to a fairly recent phenomenon in prostate cancer treatment—urologists opening up large radiation facilities to which—no surprise—they send patients they have diagnosed with localized prostate cancer.

In an article published in 2011 in *Prostate Cancer Communication: Choices,* the newsletter of the nonprofit group Patient Advocates for Advanced Cancer Treatments, Michael J. Dattoli, MD, called Urorad "an egregious scam being perpetrated upon prostate cancer patients, right under our noses and with the complicity of the federal government."

Dr. Dattoli is himself a board-certified radiation oncologist who does not have a Urorad facility, so perhaps he has another agenda, a competitive one. But his concerns have been voiced elsewhere. Medicare reimburses IMRT (intensity-modulated radiation therapy) at a much higher rate than surgery: as much as $40,000 compared with about $7,000 for a radical prostatectomy and about $1,500 for seeding, according to Dr. Dattoli's figures. He says that between 2003 and 2008, the period of time when Urorad facilities grew exponentially, reimbursements for IMRT increased by 84 percent, to $104 million.

One of the urologists I interviewed, Dr. Aaron Katz, brought up the subject himself and could barely contain his anger.

"A number of urologists around this country own these vast radiation centers," Dr. Katz says, "and they have tripled their income. They get these little Gleason 6 cases [I was one of those "little" Gleason 6s] and refer them for radiation at facilities in which they have ownership. Here they are making $45,000 and $50,000 on every little Gleason 6. Every day. Five days a week.

"These guys were dying financially. Okay, the robot comes along and maybe some got good on that, but if you're in your late 50s or early 60s, you're not going to learn robotic surgery. 'But wait a minute! I can just refer a patient for radiation, sit in my office, and collect a paycheck for the radiation center I own? Why don't I do that?'

"And people wonder why medical costs are being driven up. It makes me sick to think about it."

AS A FURTHER EXAMPLE of how complicated the prostate cancer picture can be, consider that while Dr. Katz rages about over-irradiating, he is an advocate for cryotherapy, also known as "focal ablation," a treatment that is not without controversy.

In simplest terms, cryo freezes the cancerous tissue, causing the cells to die. Dr. Katz has been doing the procedure for 20 years and, after performing 2,000 procedures and teaching more than 100 other urologist–surgeons to do it, he stands squarely behind it.

"It is an excellent modality for men who have radiation-recurrent disease, or for men who had a small area of cancer and are uncomfortable with surveillance," Dr. Katz told me. "You would've been an excellent candidate for focal ablation with your low level of cancer. It's outpatient therapy. It takes me about an hour to do with minimal anesthesia.

"It's [included] in the area of radiation, I suppose, because all radiation is ablation technology. But radiation is whole-gland treatment, while this is just focusing on the cancer, freezing the zone of the cancer shown by the biopsy."

Most everyone agrees that cryo is effective for stopping cancer. But it's the side effects that have some worried.

"I just operated on a guy yesterday who had cryotherapy," says Dr. Blaivis, "and this guy's life has been changed without any reasonable hope of a satisfactory outcome. Aaron has made an honest effort at looking at the science of it, but the complications happen later and there is always an intellectual reason to explain that it was a success. I respect Aaron's efforts, but totally disagree with his conclusions."

Dr. Van Arsdalen says much the same thing. "The side effects from cryo, especially getting a hole in the rectum, are typically worse than the side effects from radiation or surgery," he says. "They may not be common, but that doesn't mean they aren't devastating."

Dr. Lee takes a position somewhere in between.

"There are a lot of intellectual differences between doctors, and you are on thin ice when you start criticizing what other people do if you don't do the procedure yourself," says Dr. Lee. "You have to look at data and become really familiar with it before you say it is good or bad.

"Cancer cure–wise, cryo is actually pretty good. Side effect–wise, it may not be as good as other things."

A final thought: The fact that cryo is controversial does not make it wrong, particularly in the hands of someone as respected as Aaron Katz. And it is certainly not wrong because I bring it up.

I have mentioned that I am not a doctor, right?

I CONFESS THAT I HAD A HARD TIME PLUGGING IN to the ED research process. Had I flatlined (so to speak) in that department, I would've had more motivation, but my supposition all along has been that things will get back to 100 percent, or near 100 percent, with only conventional auxiliary assistance, "conventional" being defined as an ED pill. That supposition continues to this day, even though I'm at about, say, 80 percent. But that might not be how you look at it, and there are plenty of options to consider, including the permanent one of a penile prosthesis, which is, obviously, introduced surgically.

A less radical and more common plan of attack is to use the penis pump, described at one Web site as "a tried-and-true device." Well, not tried by me, although I include an anecdote about its usage among the personal stories recounted in Chapter 15. I would not recommend an Internet search if your goal is to find out the positives and negatives of the pump because there's some pretty hysterical stuff out there. One example: "The unnatural method I employed for inflating my organ has resulted in a total loss of sensation in my organ. I have almost lost all sense of touch, and that is driving my wife up the wall." Talk to your doctor about the pump. It is not some Bizarro World device. It is commonly used and, apparently, used with some degree of success.

There is also plenty of information about natural remedies for ED, including a supplement made from the bark of the yohimbe tree, an evergreen native to Africa. I wouldn't advise sending off for a year's supply of yohimbe without talking to a doctor, and, to be sure, some suggested herbal remedies are utter nonsense. But it's a legitimate area for research. MayoClinic.com, a Web site that is well within the medical mainstream, has a section on "erectile dysfunction herbs." At the same time, though, it urges caution. Here's what it says about something called epimedium, which is also known as—I'm not making this up—horny goat weed. "This traditional Chinese medicine may help erectile dysfunction, [but] there's little evidence about the safety or side effects of epimedium. It may cause blood thinning and lower blood pressure."

The one remedy I was tempted to try was MUSE. As you would suspect, MUSE has nothing to do with artistic inspiration, but rather stands for the very unartistic "medicated urethral system for erection." My friend Jeff Mohler, whose cancer and treatment profiles basically fit mine (close in age, PSA level, biopsy results, robotic prostatectomy success) had given it a try (with mixed results; he eventually stopped using it) and offered me a couple of "hits." He left the package on his back porch for me; when I retrieved it I felt like I was making a cocaine pickup.

MUSE works like this: A thin applicator is inserted into the penis. (The instructions explicitly state that the applicator is to be inserted "inside the opening at the end of the penis," though I can't imagine where else it would go other than the "opening" if it is indeed to go into the penis.) You press a button on the applicator that releases a pellet of medication, which is absorbed through the membrane that lines the inside of the urethra. The medication theoretically relaxes the muscles in the surrounding blood vessels of the penis, thus increasing blood flow into the penis and producing an erection. I say "theoretically" since I can't imagine any form of the verb "relax" having any relevance to this exercise.

I informed my wife that it was MUSE time.

"Since you couldn't manage to give yourself a Fleet enema without help," Donna said, "this I gotta see." Then she thought about it. "On second thought, I don't really have to see it. You can go this one alone."

"But the information on WebMD says—and I quote—'it's important to include your partner in your decision.'"

"Consider me included," she said, "just not involved."

"It also says—and I quote—'partners of men who have vision problems or who may have difficulty inserting the pellet can be taught.'"

"Your vision's twice as good as mine," she said. "Good luck."

I wanted to do it. I really did. But eventually I decided against it. I want to keep working at this thing. I will take my Cialis and strive to get back to 100 percent without pellets or pumps or yohimbe or horny goat. Especially without horny goat.

CHAPTER 13

...In which the author presents the many and varied opinions of the doctors he interviewed

UROLOGISTS, RADIOLOGISTS, AND SURGEONS know much more about prostate cancer than I do, and, unless you are a doctor yourself, much more than you know. During my months of research for this book, I never stumped a doctor with a question. I never had one of them say, "Hmm, I never heard of that." They keep up. They care. They know what they're doing.

But doctors are human. They are not infallible. They do not speak directly to God. If they did, they would speak with one thunderous yet soothing voice, and—trust me—they do not. They have their own prejudices and sometimes form their medical opinions based on those prejudices. They are like Italian grandmothers, each with her own recipe for the perfect tomato gravy, each convinced hers is the only way to make it, each convinced that all others are just so much *immondizia*.

So take much, but not everything, from these portraits of the doctors I interviewed, all of whom are involved, in one way or another, in the battle against prostate cancer.

Patrick Walsh, MD

Acclaimed Urologist, Surgeon, Researcher, and Author at Johns Hopkins

"I think we're going to see death rates [from prostate cancer] go back up again."

Dr. Walsh's second full-time job was as director of the Johns Hopkins Brady Urological Institute. That's something like the urological equivalent of coming out of high school and starting as shortstop for the New York Yankees. By the age of 30, Dr. Walsh, the son of an Akron, Ohio, cigar store owner, had a track record in all fields of urology, which had a long way to go in 1974, the year he took over at Hopkins.

Men were presenting at doctors' offices with advanced metastatic cancer. Radical prostatectomies were rarely performed (in only about 7 percent of diagnosed cases) because the procedure produced a gruesome amount of blood loss, permanent disappearance of sexual potency in almost every man, and permanent loss of urinary control in up to 25 percent of men. That meant there was little research and development going on because of the dearth of available post-op tissue. "Both patients and physicians agreed," said Dr. Walsh, "that the treatment was worse than the disease." Plus, radiation, the most common form of intervention, was nowhere near as sophisticated and effective as it is today.

So Dr. Walsh set out to find a better way to extract a cancerous prostate. He turned his operating room "into an anatomy lab," as he puts it, and studied cadavers of young males in whom the tissue wasn't so deformed. His *aha* moment came when he isolated the trunks of nerves that led to the prostate and those that were involved in erection. This is a vast oversimplification, of course, but the bottom line is that Dr. Walsh began performing prostatectomies that did not result in massive blood loss and went a long way toward preserving function, particularly erectile.

He still remembers the date when he performed what he considers to be the first nerve-sparing prostatectomy.

"April 26th, 1982," he says, relaxing in his Hopkins office, though, to be honest, relaxing is not a state I associate with Dr. Walsh. "I did it on a professor of business from Cleveland. Thirty years later that man has an undetectable PSA and a normal quality of life."

What Dr. Walsh did after that was just as important—he opened the doors of his OR. "I never felt competitive about it," says Dr. Walsh. "Look, why is Hopkins on this earth? To train leaders in urology, make discoveries, and share them with others. I would ask prospective patients if they wanted to bring along their urologist so I could teach them. I've had 20 urologists in the room at one time observing me during the operation. Probably 3,000 to 4,000 have watched over these 30 years. I've made 50,000 DVDs and given them to every urologist in the world who wanted one."

(He even gave one to me. I am thinking about trying to do this radical prostatectomy thing in my spare time.)

As the number of operations went up, so did the amount of tissue available for study. With the advent of PSA testing, by the mid-1990s more and more men were being treated earlier, and better, for prostate cancer. Public awareness of and education about the disease increased exponentially, and did so again when in 2001 Dr. Walsh wrote his *Guide to Surviving Prostate Cancer*, now in its third edition.

Like many others, Dr. Walsh is angry that the USPSTF never contacted him for input, but positively aggrieved at what he sees as the deleterious effects that will result from the recommendation against PSA screening.

"What I worry about are the young men who are listening to the advice that they shouldn't get tested," says Dr. Walsh. "In 1990, 20 percent of men who were newly diagnosed with prostate cancer had metastases to bone. That's just a fact. Now it's 3 percent. If you take the death rate from prostate cancer in 1990 and the most recent data in 2008, the number should be about 60,000 deaths. But it's only 28,000 deaths. Why?

"Because we improved the surgical procedures and PSA [tests] came along. Now it's easier for us to find the men who are curable, and suddenly, we have what we had in most other fields of medicine—a way to diagnose the disease at a curable stage and a curative form of treatment. And what results is a tremendous decline in mortality.

"But if people listen to the USPSTF, I think we're going to see death rates go back up again. With the influx of the baby boomers, [by 2050] there's going to be about 40 million men in the age group that's most susceptible to prostate cancer.

"Plus, men are living longer. Between 1975 and 2000, deaths from cardiovascular disease in men under the age of 85 fell by about 50 percent. They used to say that people didn't die from prostate cancer because they will die from something else. But now people are living longer and not dying of cardiovascular disease. And so they will die of prostate cancer."

James Manley, DO
My Primary Care Physician

"We have to look at patients on an individual basis."

I have been going to Dr. Manley for almost 20 years. We've grown older together. I feel like I know him even though we don't socialize outside of the office. He probably feels like he knows me, too. Oh, the anatomical secrets that a PCP takes to the grave.

When I interview him, he gives me his thoughts on primary care philosophy and the USPSTF recommendations against testing.

"No matter what the panel says, it is putting a much greater emphasis on cost than we ever had before," says Dr. Manley. "It is about numbers. How many people do I have to put on a statin to prevent one heart attack? How many people do I have to order a PSA test for to prevent one death from prostate cancer? And all the statistics in the world can't hide this fact: If you happen to be the one in a hundred or the one in a thousand who dies from something because you were not screened, the numbers don't mean anything to you.

"The controversy is only going to get worse, and I think primary care doctors are really going to have to look at the reasoning behind these recommendations against screenings. Let's say a man comes to me at age 50 and I don't recommend PSA screening, and at 55 he comes back with lower-back pain and it turns out to be prostate cancer. And he wants to sue me because I did not order a PSA test. I can say, 'Well, they told me not to screen.' Okay, we'll see if lawyers really care about that."

Dr. Manley pulls up the USPSTF recommendations on his smartphone and begins reading.

"Okay, 55-year-old, doesn't smoke, sexually active. The 'A' recommendations include aspirin to prevent cardiovascular disease. Colon cancer screening gets an A. High blood pressure screening, an A. That makes sense.

"But then how ridiculous is this? HIV screening and syphilis screening are also A recommendations. Really? Where are they getting the numbers from? I have been in practice for 25 years and I have never—never—had a newly diagnosed HIV patient."

"That's because you serve, basically, a white, suburban, middle-class population," I say.

"That's exactly my point," says Dr. Manley. "Individual doctors should decide what screens are necessary and what are not. And I am still waiting for one of these higher-up, ivory-tower docs to convince me that we will do worse in the long run by testing somebody as opposed to [seeing] someone to whom we do nothing and his cancer eventually metastasizes. They try to tell me that the average man is going to die of something else. Well, not somebody who gets prostate cancer at 40. That guy is going to die of prostate cancer if he's not treated."

Dr. Manley believes that the USPSTF guidelines are more about future cost considerations than about the tests themselves. That may be obvious. According to the Web site Healthcare Blue Book, a PSA test costs between $23 and $45. But that turns into at least $1,500 if it leads to biopsy at an ambulatory surgery center. The digital rectal exam doesn't cost anything (unless you want to add up the damage done over time to a physician's finger, or a patient's psyche), yet it gets a D rating, just like the PSA test. What could be the harm in doing a test that literally takes seconds and just might uncover something?

"What they're worried about is not the cost of the test, but the costs that can result when something is discovered because of the test," he says.

Dr. Manley understands the general movement toward eliminating screening tests that might be ineffective. And he believes the common wisdom that younger primary care physicians, schooled in an era when the USPSTF has a heavy hand in health care, will be far less likely to screen for anything that is not rated A or B. But in his 25th year of practice, he's not about to do a one-eighty on prostate cancer.

"When I train younger physicians," says Dr. Manley, "I still tell them the old-fashioned way—PSA screening and digital rectal exams. As a family doctor, my primary goal is to keep people living healthy lives for as long as possible. To do that, we have to look at patients on an individual basis. Right now I have a patient who is in his mid-70s. He swims a mile a day, walks the course every time he plays golf. He is in better shape than some 20-year-olds I see. He had prostate cancer, he wanted it out, and I agreed. Why not? He has an excellent chance of living 20 more years, so why not give him every opportunity to do that? But a person his age with dementia? Of course not. You don't treat him. You don't give him radiation.

"As for you, I would recommend exactly what we did. I still think a healthy young person—and I'm going to consider you young in this case—has a better chance at longevity by getting the cancer out. That is not going to change for me."

Jerry Blaivas, MD
Noted New York City Urologist

"I consider myself an agnostic when it comes to prostate cancer."

Several years ago, when Dr. Blaivas was being treated for a kidney stone, a couple of residents, without telling him, made sure that his PSA was checked in routine blood work. Smiling all the while, they told him what the reading was. He doesn't remember the number (it wasn't high), but he does remember his annoyance.

"They did it as a joke, but I didn't appreciate it," says Dr. Blaivas. "Things like that have very serious consequences."

Dr. Blaivas is a clinical professor of urology at Weill Cornell Medical College, an attending surgeon at NewYork-Presbyterian and Lenox Hill Hospitals, and the father-in-law of a friend of mine, Chris Stone, the managing editor of *Sports Illustrated*. Chris told me to be sure to interview him.

"Jerry's a smart guy with a lot of opinions," said Chris.

Right on both counts.

Dr. Blaivas's specialty is not prostate cancer. It is treating bladder-related complications resulting from urological treatment, incontinence in particular. Dr. Aaron Katz calls Dr. Blaivas "the father of urodynamics, one of the important people who invented testing for men and women with bladder issues." Along the way, Dr. Blaivas has developed some strong opinions about prostate cancer.

Or, looking at it another way, he hasn't come to any opinion at all.

"I consider myself an agnostic when it comes to prostate cancer," Dr. Blaivas tells me at his office on the Upper East Side of Manhattan. "Most urologists believe that prostate cancer is a deadly disease and that early detection and treatment is of benefit. I'm an agnostic on that point. It has yet to be proven to my satisfaction.

"If prostate cancer could be cured by a pill with no side effects, there would be no controversy. Or if treatment killed 90 percent of the patients, there would be no controversy. But we're in the middle of that.

"And the middle is this: Most 62-year-old men [with] Gleason 6 [he's talking about me here] would live out a normal life expectancy whether or not they're treated."

Keep in mind, as Dr. Blaivas himself acknowledges, that he is coming at this from the perspective of someone who sees symptoms that result from treatment. He doesn't usually see men dying of prostate cancer; instead, he sees men with issues related to prostate cancer intervention, both surgical and radiological.

"You might say that makes me biased because I see so many complications," he says. "And, yes, I see that downside all the time. But what I'm saying is that we don't even know if the upside is curative. So for me, it's just not worth it."

I ask him if he would advise his son-in-law, my friend, to get a PSA test.

"No," says Dr. Blaivas. "I would advise my son-in-law to be aware of colon cancer, glaucoma, blood pressure, and diabetes. About those things I am not an agnostic. I'm on the bandwagon. Those things, we know that if you're screened and diagnosed early the treatment is unequivocal. That's not the case for prostate cancer.

"My big public education push, if I can call it that, is whether to get screened in the first place. To me, that's the crucial decision a person makes. Because unless you're really in the know about it, the odds are overwhelming that you will end up with a prostate biopsy if you have an elevated PSA. And there's a pretty good chance that you'll end up with prostate cancer and a pretty good chance that you'll end up with treatment that could've been avoided if you had never gotten screening in the first place."

I ask him if he agrees with the USPSTF recommendation against PSAs. That puts him in a tough spot. Doctors as a whole are reflexively against government intrusion, and Dr. Blaivas will give you chapter and verse on the consequences of having too many federal rules and regulations.

"I think people should at the very least become as educated about their health as they are about anything else in life," answers Dr. Blaivas. "Most guys know more about the details of what car they're going to buy or what sports team they follow than they know about their health. Much as you did. You investigated. You talked to people."

But I wouldn't have known about my prostate cancer, I tell him, without my primary care physician telling me that I had an elevated PSA.

"I'm not saying you or your doctor did anything wrong," answers Dr. Blaivas. "What I am saying is that I would've preferred he sat you down and told you all about prostate screening."

Dr. Blaivas makes it clear that he would never tell me I made a mistake by having surgery. (Or tell me that outright, anyway.) And he allows that deciding on intervention, if it comes to that, is a personal decision that might involve extenuating factors.

"All the men in my family died of cardiovascular disease, diabetes, things like that," says Dr. Blaivas. "One hundred percent. So I figure my mortality is more heavily weighted in that direction."

I tell him that it's the opposite for me—cancer wins out over cardiovascular disease.

"That is totally understandable," he says. "Remember, I said I am an agnostic. I'm not against anything. I'm just not sure.

"And let me be clear that I have great respect for the prostate cancer treatment advocates. As a group they are incredibly bright, highly motivated, and wonderfully good surgeons. So if it's just a matter of patient preference, most people feel uncomfortable knowing there's cancer in their body. Plus, there are people for whom treatment is surely lifesaving.

"But the present data doesn't give me enough confidence to say that it's necessary or worthwhile to pursue early diagnosis and treatment. What I'm saying is that I'm older than you, and it's entirely possible that I have prostate cancer." He sends me off with a warm smile. "I just haven't checked."

Peter Bach, MD

Writer and Researcher on Cancer
and Public Health Policy

"Screening is a very,
very inefficient enterprise."

It is the worst of interview beginnings.

I meet Dr. Bach at a restaurant in Midtown Manhattan. We shake hands, we sit down, and I say:

"How is your wife? Is she doing okay?"

He pauses for a moment. "She passed away. In January of this year."

Dr. Bach had come to my attention through a series of well-written articles he had done for the *New York Times*. Some of them mentioned prostate cancer, but they were more about general health care policy, research on which he is actively involved at the national level.

He had also written about his wife, who was battling breast cancer, and I had assumed that she was still alive. I met with him in June of 2012, and at that point he hadn't been able to bring himself to write about her death. As of March 2013, he still hadn't.

Dr. Bach has written extensively about overtesting in medicine. He was part of that chorus telling me that I had probably done the wrong thing in opting for surgery. But he was telling me so eloquently. So in what seemed like a logical segue, I asked if his wife, Ruth, who had been 46 when she died, had received regular mammograms.

"It is perfectly okay to ask me that question," says Dr. Bach. "But I have decided I'm not going to answer it. I'll tell you my reason. Obviously it's not privacy, because I've written about her illness. My worry is that people will look at individual cases and ask those sorts of questions and make judgments. If I say that she was 43 and had regular mammographies, one would conclude, 'Oh, they must not work very well.' And if I said she didn't get them, some might conclude, 'Oh, how irresponsible. That's the reason she died.'"

We discuss his general feelings about what he considers over-screening in medicine. I have my speech prepared:

"It would seem to me, Dr. Bach," I say, "that part of my medical knowledge about myself should include whether or not I have cancer."

"I understand that," he says. "I really do. But screening in general is a very, very inefficient enterprise. You have to understand the math. I don't even have to talk about prostate cancer. Take breast cancer. You have to screen about 1,000 women between [the ages of] 40 and 50 for 10 years to prevent one breast cancer death. That's a very, very inefficient thing to do.

"Now, for prostate cancer, if you look at the trials—and this was with people with worse prostate cancer than you had—the difference in prostate mortality between those who were screened and those who weren't was about 4 percent. Everything in health care is about probability." (You also have to understand that "everything in health care" is about different interpretations of studies, which is the case here.)

"I understand that," I say. "But isn't there a difference between overtesting and overtreatment? Whether or not I get treated might be a difficult decision. But whether or not I have cancer seems to be something an individual should know."

"Why?" asks Dr. Bach.

That stops me for a moment. "Well, for the same reason you want to know if you have a cold," I answer. (I'm a really skilled debater.)

"Well, I don't necessarily want useless knowledge," Dr. Bach says. "Do you want to know what software your broker is using to manage your stocks?"

"I'd have to say that's not the same thing," I answer.

He thinks about that. "I guess I agree it's not the same thing. But what you'd want to know about your broker is things that affect your planning, your financial future. You don't need to know everything."

Dr. Bach says that some screening interventions are worthwhile. "We found out that if you take a tongue depressor and scrape off cells from a woman's cervix, it is a very accurate screen for cervical cancer. Cervical cancer death rates have dropped, like, 90 percent. We all but got rid of it. It's fantastic. But other screening tests just don't work as well."

Dr. Bach does say that family history matters. Yet though his own father—Fritz Bach, MD, a celebrated physician and researcher who helped develop techniques that enable people to better survive organ and bone marrow transplants—had prostate cancer, Peter does not agonize about getting a PSA test. "My father had radiation and recovered just fine from prostate cancer," he says. "He died of a heart attack. It [the PSA test] is just something I don't worry about too much. Once every 10 years I get my cholesterol checked. I get my blood pressure checked every once in a while. And maybe I could stand to lose a few pounds. But I don't need a doctor to tell me that."

His position is that medical science errs by vast commission and almost never by omission. And he's sticking with that opinion. But he doesn't want me to feel depressed about having had surgery.

"Look, that idea of getting something early, stopping it in its tracks, being aggressive," says Dr. Bach, "is very potent logic. The problem is, it's not biology.

"But I'll give you this much: Think of it as a seat belt analogy. I assume you wear a seat belt, and I have been wearing one ever since I started driving even though I haven't had an accident in 20 years. So apparently I'm over–seat belting. But of course I'm not."

"So what I did when I had surgery," I tell Dr. Bach, "is the urological equivalent of over–seat belting."

"A good way to put it," he says.

Keith Van Arsdalen, MD
My Friend and Urologist

"You were too young and too healthy for active surveillance."

During the two years that Keith and I intersected as fraternity brothers at Muhlenberg College four decades ago, the subject of urology, needless to say, never came up. Neither did most serious subjects unless you consider the fate of our intramural football team, which was in fact quite serious. Everyone knew that Keith would become a doctor, and a good one, but there was not much chatter about specialties.

"I didn't know myself what field I wanted to get into," says Keith. "I had a couple of rotations [at the Medical College of Virginia] that I didn't like, but when I got to urology I was with a bunch of guys who were really fun. We really hit it off. At first, it had as much to do with that as anything. But as I got further in to it, the field turned out to be fascinating. There were so many aspects to it."

Keith came to Penn to do research on the relationship between spinal cord injury and voiding dysfunction. Gradually, he branched out into the general area of urodynamics and then he became an expert in stones. (We were interested in Stones in college, although they were the Rolling variety.) Through it all, though, Keith was never far from prostate cancer.

And he says that what he sees these days compared to what he saw 30 years ago has convinced him that PSA screening is a good thing.

"We used to have our own ward here, maybe 35 beds, and at least half of them, sometimes the entire ward, consisted of older men with metastatic prostate cancer," says Keith. "They were going to die. They were here with these huge prostate cancers that kept them from urinating, with bone pain, with all sorts of problems.

"But when someone comes in these days and presents with those symptoms, we say, 'Oh, my God.' Because we just don't see them anymore. So when people say we shouldn't do any screening, I say that while statistics might show we haven't altered life expectancy dramatically, we also don't have a ward full of people with metastatic disease.

"Why? Because the cancer is being found earlier. And there is no other conclusion I can reach except that it's the PSA test that made that difference. So for me it's still worthwhile doing the screening. The mortality might not be different. But the morbidity certainly is."

Having said that, Keith does concede that he looked at me differently in 2011 than he would've in 1981 or even 2001. Although he crossed active surveillance off my list of reasonable options back in September 2011, he says he is comfortable with it in certain circumstances.

"I had a patient in here this week," says Keith. "He's 69. He's got 1 core with 20 percent cancer out of 14 cores. He's a Gleason 6. Negative bone scan. PSA of 4.2 and a list of medical problems a foot long.

"If it were me, I would choose active surveillance in that case. At the very least—or I should say at the most—I would choose radiation. Why should he have a radical procedure with all the attendant risk—even just the anesthesia—for a cancer that probably won't kill him and he has so many other problems?

"But no matter what I say, he wants a radical prostatectomy. He wants the robot. It's his choice and I can't talk him out of it. What a doctor must do is present the options in the most realistic way possible. But it's up to the patient to decide."

So, I ask him, why didn't he favor active surveillance for me?

He thinks about that for a moment and answers this way:

"A doctor must develop a sense of how he's going to counsel patients. I can't counsel you differently because I know you. So you develop parameters that fit most people.

"None of this is simple, so I'm not going to say it's simple. But I thought you were too young to do active surveillance. I felt that sooner or later you would have to be treated for prostate cancer.

"Can I say that with certainty? No. At this point, there is no other test we can do that looks at the characteristics of the cancer and says definitively that this will be the type that will kick into gear and metastasize. I wish we could determine that."

I tell him the anecdote of one doctor waving my report in the air and scoffing about the low level of cancer. (See Aaron Katz, MD, page 124.) Keith responds, "Let's say you were 55. It would not be unreasonable to say, 'Okay, I'm going to take five years of watching, buy those five years when I don't have potency or incontinence issues, and maybe get treated when I'm 60.' To that, I would probably say fine.

"At the same time I don't think it's an unreasonable assumption that the cancer is going to grow. It wasn't 2 percent de novo. [You gotta love a urologist with a Latin background.] It started at half a percent, then 1 percent, then 2, then 3. Maybe it started when you were 40 and it took 20 years to get there. Now, in another 20 years maybe it wouldn't have grown. But maybe it would have.

"So given that uncertainty, I felt comfortable advising intervention. And it would've been the same for any patient with your parameters."

John Christodouleas, MD

Radiation Oncologist, Penn Medicine

"We need to change the culture surrounding the PSA."

Had I chosen radiation, I would've chosen Dr. C., whose name I have shortened throughout this book to both save me the extra characters and reduce the chances of errant typing. Radiation oncologists sometimes remain outside the tight circle of prostate treatment decisions since they generally are not urologists, the first doctors whom prostate patients see. At Penn, though, Dr. C. seems to be part of the team, and he keeps up with every development in prostate cancer treatment.

He is not a prostate agnostic, as Dr. Blaivas is, but neither is he a standard-bearer for PSA screening. And he is certainly more willing than many to embrace active surveillance.

"The data is getting stronger and stronger that you probably don't need to do anything for a very large percentage of patients," says Dr. C. "Look, I was trained in the Hopkins tradition and influenced by Bal Carter. They have the age of 65 as the line. That is very conservative, and there is more and more data to suggest that any man with low-risk prostate cancer is very unlikely to develop problems. So I would say over the last 10 years I've gotten more and more comfortable with active surveillance."

"You mean for patients like myself?" I ask.

"Yes, like you," says Dr. C., who, if you'll recall, had my records and did examine me.

"Do you agree with the USPSTF recommendations against the PSA test?" I ask him.

"I wouldn't say I agree with them," says Dr. C., "but I would say that the rationale they used—to try to limit overtreatment—is correct. Yes, we've identified the problem, which is: Lots of people die of prostate cancer. But is the solution lots of PSA screening? That's a more difficult question.

"If I told you that getting PSA screening increases your chance of living six months longer by 3 percent, is it worth screening every man in this country? I'm not saying I know the answer to that question. I'm just saying that it's very reasonable to ask.

"Now, throwing away PSA screening entirely is throwing the baby out with the bathwater. But if we were able to develop a culture of not overinterpreting the PSA, then maybe we could have our cake and eat it, too. People have skin cancers all the time, and they don't start rewriting their wills. The doctor says, 'Ah, it's a little skin cancer.' That happens all the time.

"But that view of being able to preserve the PSA but change the culture around it? Many people think that's naïve. You can't have something that a lot of men die of and try to explain that 97 percent, maybe higher, don't die of it. It's hard for patients not to get scared, particularly when you have a health care system that is driven by action."

Aaron Katz, MD

Chairman of Urology,
Winthrop-University Hospital

"You take away biopsies . . . you'll go back to the day when the main thing urologists are doing is treating clap."

We are at a Japanese restaurant in Garden City, Long Island, across the street from Winthrop-University Hospital, and Dr. Katz will have the sushi, as he does three times a week.

Dr. Katz is not a completely unconventional urologist. He opposes the USPSTF recommendations about PSAs and typically orders screening for his patients because he considers it a helpful diagnostic tool. He does operate for prostate cancer, with his intervention specialty being cryotherapy (see Chapter 12).

But he also has an alternative medicine bent, which he prefers to label "integrative medicine." Before he came to Winthrop, he was the director of the Center for Holistic Urology at Columbia University

Medical Center. The general philosophy there involved combining diet, herbal medicines, lifestyle changes, and stress management with more conventional treatments to figure out what was best for the patient. That specialty began when he studied with Robert Atkins, MD—yes, that Dr. Atkins. To be clear, Dr. Katz tells me he is not an advocate of the Atkins praise-the-protein-and-pass-the-pork-chop diet. But he does advocate, as did Dr. Atkins, the concept of integrating other factors into traditional treatment.

"There is no section of the AUA [American Urological Association] just on integrative medicine," says Dr. Katz. "There is a board of doctors interested in alternative medicine, and I have started my own Society of Integrative Urology, the SIU. I'm hoping to gain greater acceptance by the AUA and urologists."

Dr. Katz's most celebrated patient is media personality Don Imus, who has elected to deal with his prostate cancer with diet, herbal medicine, and supplements. Dr. Katz has appeared on Imus's morning simulcast show (full disclosure: so have I, though to talk about basketball, not the prostate) to discuss alternative prostate cancer treatments.

"When I go and talk around the country," says Dr. Katz, "I can't believe the number who want more information about this. When we did a survey, [we found that more than] 70 percent of urologists would use more of these treatments if they knew more. There has to be an education process surrounding this."

The direction of our conversation leads me to believe that, were he my urologist, he would not have advised intervention, whether surgical or radiological (though he may have suggested cryo).

"Okay, you had a PSA under 10, right?" he says.

"Well under 10," I say.

"You do not have a family history of prostate cancer?"

"Colon cancer."

"Doesn't matter. You're not African American, obviously."

"Obviously," I say.

"You had a slow-rising PSA and a biopsy that showed a Gleason 6. What did your MRI show?"

"That the cancer was contained in the gland," I answer.

He looks at me and spreads his hands. He has made his opinion clear. I told him that I was leaning in that direction when I got the word from Dr. Carter at Hopkins that I would be too young for his study.

"Well, that doesn't mean that active surveillance is wrong for a guy who's 62 years old or even 45 years old," answers Dr. Katz. "It just means that Bal Carter decided to cut it off there because he doesn't want to start saying, 'At Hopkins, we don't do anything at age 50.' It's a little more tolerable, a little more acceptable, not to do anything at age 65."

Then I show Dr. Katz my postsurgical pathology report. He studies it for a moment and cups both his hands around his mouth as if to shout to the entire restaurant.

"Oh, my God! Gland involvement, 2 percent. Let's operate on this guy. He has cancer! Get him into surgery right away!"

It's a light moment. I laugh. He laughs.

"The actual pathology said 'between 2 and 10 percent,'" I say. "But I guess you believe I made the wrong decision."

"I never go back in time," says Dr. Katz. "I only go forward with my patients. You thought about what you were getting done and, fortunately, it sounds like you hit the trifecta. Your PSA is zero, right? You are continent, right? And you are potent enough for intercourse without Viagra or Cialis, right?"

"Well, all of those except maybe, kind of, sort of, the last one," I say. "But I'm working on it."

"Okay. You made the decision that you considered right for you, so therefore it's right for you. You saw the right surgeon. You're moving on. You're writing a book, which is in some ways cathartic.

"I hope I'm not coming across as negative. There's a lot of good doctors out there. Great urologists, great surgeons. And some men have aggressive prostate cancer. Men need to be treated. Men die of the disease, men with Gleasons of 8 and 9, high PSAs, MRIs showing cancer outside the prostate.

"But for the majority of men whose PSAs went from 3 to 4, small area of cancer, Gleason 6? Those men should be strongly offered— I don't care what age—the idea of watching and waiting. Because why take a 45-year-old guy and subject him to surgery when even in the best of hands that guy could lose his erections forever? Yeah, you may have 'cured' him, so to speak. But he may never have normal sexual relations again and will never experience ejaculation."

One of Dr. Katz's ideas is to change the Gleason system, perhaps to not even allow Gleason 6s to appear on the scale and to give a new name to cancers such as mine.

"Right away guys in your position think of the friend who died of pancreatic cancer," says Dr. Katz. "Or my son who had an aggressive leukemia and whose life was on the line." (His son has recovered.)

So what should we call it?

"Call it 'atypical' or 'preneoplastic,'" Dr. Katz suggests. "Anything but 'cancer.' Because in one sense you don't really have prostate cancer. You have some abnormal cells in your prostate, and the risk of it getting out of the prostate is extremely low."

Dr. Katz's final target is Dr. Catalona, whom he refers to, pejoratively, as "Mr. PSA."

"If you talk to Bill Catalona, he'll say everybody needs a PSA, everybody needs a biopsy, everybody needs a prostatectomy," says Dr. Katz. "And you know what? The AUA loves this guy. All he wants to do is biopsy and operate, biopsy and operate. So the AUA makes money. It's business. Cancer is big business. You take away biopsies, you take away a lot of prostate cancer, and—whoa!—next thing you know you'll go back to the day when the main thing urologists are doing is treating clap."

Well, let's let Mr. PSA address those comments himself.

William Catalona, MD
God of the PSA Test

"As far as active surveillance goes . . . it's becoming like apple pie and motherhood."

The photographs in Dr. Catalona's office, located in Northwestern University's Feinberg School of Medicine just off Chicago's Magnificent Mile, are a notch or two above the predictable. There he is at Yankee Stadium, wearing a Yankees cap and posing with then-manager Joe Torre. Torre was his patient. There is Dr. Catalona with baseball immortal Stan Musial, who died in January 2013. Musial was a patient. There he is with Syracuse basketball coach Jim Boeheim. Boeheim was a patient.

There's a signed photo of the late Yankees owner George Steinbrenner. Was he a patient? "I can't say," says Dr. Catalona. Ditto for boxer Gene Tunney, another photo subject. There is Dr. Catalona with Senator Robert Dole. Dole was not a patient, but they became acquainted on the prostate cancer circuit. "The first time I ever met Senator Dole, he said to me, 'Thanks for saving my life, Doctor,'" says Catalona. "I never forgot that."

Dr. Catalona is synonymous with the PSA test. In the late 1980s he was at a meeting with a group of other urologists. "The specific goal of that meeting was to lower the death rate of prostate cancer by [the year] 2000," Dr. Catalona remembers. "There were all sorts of ideas, some of them wild. I remember there was a Japanese doctor who came up with an ultrasound probe on a toilet seat. Men would sit on it and that would test for prostate cancer. 'That may fly in Japan,' I told the guy, 'but it's not going to go over here.'"

Dr. Catalona says an idea suddenly came to him during a jog on the beach when he was at the conference: Use the PSA test—which at that time was used purely as a marker of cancer progression—as a screening test. Though he hadn't officially studied it, he firmly believed that men with more advanced cancers at the time of surgery tended to have the highest PSA levels. The idea would be to catch the cancer early, when something might be done about it.

"I had been doing PSA testing on all my patients: BPH patients, normal patients, prostate cancer patients," Dr. Catalona tells me. "I thought it might work. So I stood up and said, 'I think the PSA test would be a good test for prostate cancer.' And I got howled down.

"See, what everyone was looking for was something like a pregnancy test. Positive you have it, negative you don't. We all knew that some men with high PSAs didn't have prostate cancer, and some had cancer with low PSAs. So everyone rejected the idea.

"But then I suggested establishing the cutoff at 4. If a man had a PSA of 4 or above, he should have a biopsy for prostate cancer. I felt the PSA was more reliable than the rectal exam, the ultrasound, or anything else."

Most everyone shrugged, he says. But Dr. Catalona organized a study that included 1,653 patients and concluded that PSA testing detected cancer several years earlier than a DRE and could be used as a screening test. His research appeared in the April 25, 1991, issue of the *New England Journal of Medicine*, and William Catalona became a medical sensation. He didn't rise to the level of Jonas Salk, Alexander Fleming, Christiaan Barnard, or Michael DeBakey, but he was featured in a *Time* magazine article, made the rounds of the morning talk shows, and became known throughout the urological world.

It took a while for the proposal to wend its way to FDA approval, but in 1994 the agency recommended the PSA test as "an aid to the early detection of prostate cancer in men who had a PSA between 4 and 10."

Dr. Catalona's research continued for 12 years, with the number of subjects reaching 36,000, and eventually his statistics showed that the PSA cutoff should be reduced to 2.5. Because of Dr. Catalona, prostate cancer is rarely found when PSA testing is not involved, and he says he firmly believes that "the prostate cancer death rate has come down by 44 percent in this country as a result of PSA testing."

You know what the USPSTF says to that: The percentage of lives saved does not compensate for the deleterious effects of biopsy and intervention. On the other hand, the majority of doctors and medical experts I talked to agree that PSA has saved lives.

Whatever your feelings about PSA, I've come to believe that the same thing Dr. Catalona says about robotic surgery—that it has been oversold—can be said about the PSA test. It is not "a simple blood test that can detect prostate cancer," as is so often stated. Instead, I would give it this definition: "The PSA is a simple and inexpensive blood test that has a good chance of identifying prostate cancer. But it may also indicate other conditions such as BPH, and, in doing so, throw off mixed signals that result in confusion, angst, and, quite possibly, over-treatment. The results of PSA tests should be combined with serious conversations with a primary care physician and/or a urologist to determine the best course of treatment."

I ask Dr. Catalona if he has changed his treatment philosophy at all after five decades in practice. He doesn't answer yes or no, but makes it clear that he knows he is the target of anti-PSA crusaders, that he's considered in some quarters to be a dinosaur clinging to an out-of-date philosophy.

"It's become the party line that there is too much overtreatment," says Dr. Catalona, "but there's no real evidence for that. And as far as active surveillance goes, yes, more and more people are pushing for it. It's becoming like apple pie and motherhood. Well, it's not as much fun as people think. First of all, there is no way you can accurately tell which patients have harmless prostate cancer. You consider only one or two cores and PSA density, and you're still wrong a third of the time.

"And you're supposed to get biopsied every year or every other year. For a patient with a long life expectancy, that's too many biopsies."

Dr. Catalona is 70, but he continues to see patients, teach, operate, research, and offer up his convictions without evincing a sliver of doubt. "I'm glad you came out well from your robotic surgery," he says as he escorts me out of his office, "but I still would've advised you that the open procedure would've been best." And as I concluded the writing of this book, I was still receiving e-mails from him touting the open surgery method.

David Lee, MD
My Surgeon

"When guys get diagnosed with late-stage prostate cancer, it's the urologists, not the researchers, who have to tell them, 'Sorry, Mr. Jones. We caught this too late.'"

I am a golfer, but not one of those types who tell you that profound truths about character and the meaning of life are learned on the course. But after playing a couple rounds with Dr. Lee, I did get insight into the way he performs as a surgeon. He will not deviate from his pre-shot routine. He will not address the ball until he's ready. He will not be distracted. He is precise in his movements. He hits the ball with the same takeaway and follow-through every time. He is scrupulous about observing the rules and rituals of the game.

Performing a robotic prostatectomy is a technical achievement.

Those who become great at it do so only after repetition, by making the same movements, following the same procedures, observing the sacred rituals of nerve sparing. After thousands of robotic prostatectomies, Dr. Lee is a bit of a robot himself, and that is intended as a compliment.

He performs between 8 and 10 prostatectomies per week, each procedure helping to pay for those two $1.9 million da Vinci robots at Penn Presbyterian in the hope that Dr. Lee will cure patients and make that cash register sing. He still sees patients, but mostly for brief introductions and post-op follow-ups. He does not do many DREs these days, does not even write many prescriptions since his PAs can handle that.

And that made me wonder if he has become divorced from the underpinnings of his profession, the day-to-day research and controversy that dogs this nettlesome subject of prostate cancer.

That answer is no.

"I feel very involved in this whole controversy, because the group that feels most strongly about prostate cancer, screening, saving lives, and preventing side effects is urologists," says Dr. Lee. "That's what I am above all. Urologists are the people who have to deal with cancer very directly. When guys get diagnosed with late-stage prostate cancer, it's the urologists, not the researchers, who have to tell them, 'Sorry, Mr. Jones. We caught this too late.'

"Before PSA screening started, one of the more common presentations was guys walking in symptomatic with back pain, meaning the cancer had already spread to the spine. [Once] PSA screening started, that scenario has almost gone away. But with the task force recommendation, all of us in the profession are afraid we're going to go back to those days."

Dr. Lee already offered his opinion (in Chapter 12) that, yes, biopsies can be dangerous. I ask him if death from surgery, permanent loss of sexual function, and urological difficulties are reasonable deterrents to intervention, which is the position of the USPSTF.

"I've seen them talk about death from surgery being 1 in every 200, and that is absolutely ridiculous," he says. "Maybe 25 years ago, but definitely not now.

"As far as continence goes, guys do really, really well. Certainly there are exceptions, but across the population, continence returns. The ED part is definitely not as consistent.

"The crime of the Preventive Services recommendation is that they pin all the negative consequences on whether or not you're even going to get detected. They're basically telling you to put your head in the sand and say, 'I don't want to know anything.' The more reasonable approach is, get your PSAs, get your biopsy if you need it, find out what your Gleason is, then make an informed decision. Because I guarantee that if people stop getting PSAs we're going to miss Gleason 7s, 8s, and 9s, and that is serious."

Which brings this around to my case. Gleason 6 (that had later progressed to a Gleason 7). Localized. Near that active-surveillance border of age 65. Should I have had surgery? Wouldn't it be safe to assume, I ask Dr. Lee, that I would not have died of prostate cancer? And if so, could the argument be made that I should not have been biopsied in the first place?

He thinks about that for a moment.

"You could make that argument," he says finally. "But this is cancer. Even the Gleason 6s can make a lot of progress and start hurting people over time. And how do you know what you are until you get a PSA? Okay, you had that level of cancer and you made a decision. Another guy who's 50-some years old [might delay] getting his PSA and come up with a Gleason 8 on the biopsy. If that guy doesn't get treated in the next two or three years, he's probably going to die. And even in the population between 65 and 75, we still want to pick out those guys with aggressive disease because surgery will have a positive impact.

"I am certain that the USPSTF recommendation against PSA testing can have serious, damaging effects."

Damaging economic effects for Dr. Lee, too. Several years ago he did 480 robotic prostatectomies in one year, but in 2012, the number dwindled to 420. "I have no doubt it's a direct result of the task force," says Dr. Lee. "I worry about the guys we might be missing."

Take it for what it is. Dr. Lee is a surgeon. His medical philosophy, his estimable reputation, and his bank account have been forged, by and large, behind the controls of a robot.

But I can only say this about him: I trusted him with nothing less than my life, and I would trust him with the lives of my sons and my grandson. There's not much higher compliment you can give a man than that.

CHAPTER 14

... In which the author talks to a golfing immortal and a Viagra pioneer and ruminates on other celebrities who have died from prostate cancer, as well as others who are living with it

GOLF WASN'T MUCH OF A MANLY SPORT until Arnold Palmer came along in the mid-1950s. He stalked around the golf course like a hunter in search of big game, attacking the course more than playing it; sneered at seemingly impossible shots, stepped up to the ball, flicked away his cigarette, took a vicious weekend-golfer flail at the ball, and watched it sail inevitably greenward. He won 62 PGA tournaments and was even more dashing in the ones he lost. His Marlboro Man persona helped to sell golf, which can be a soul-crushing bore, to the masses and to television.

Do you want to watch a small ball hit in the air by a bunch of guys who look like insurance agents?

No, but we could always watch Arnie. Women loved him; men wanted to be him.

Count my father among them. He took me to see Arnie—everybody called him that, for a Marlboro Man can't have a handle like Arnold—play an exhibition match near our home in New Jersey, right around the time that Dad was teaching me the game. Jack McCallum Sr. was infatuated, as were millions of others, by Arnie's common-man ambience, his balls-out confidence, his bravado, his ability to convey the idea that you didn't have to belong to a country club to be a golfer.

And so my father would've given anything to be with me when I interviewed Arnie at his office at Bay Hill Club and Lodge, the resort he owns in Orlando, Florida, a place where the top pros still come by just to converse with the man they call the King. Though the 84-year-old Palmer sometimes pauses between words and thoughts, he remembers everything about his prostate cancer, which was diagnosed in 1997.

"When that PSA test came out, my doctor recommended it right away," says Palmer. "We did it every year from the beginning. My belief is that you should always know everything about your personal health.

"My readings started at zero, went up to 1, then 2, then 3, and when it reached 4, my doctor said, 'That's the point when you get it checked.' So they did six cores on one biopsy. I tell you what, that's no fun. Then they did six more the next year. Nothing. Then they did six more the next year. And finally they found it. The third year, they found it.

CHAPTER 14

"When I found out, I was in San Diego at a PGA tour event. 'Arn, I'm sorry to tell you,' my doctor said when he called me, 'but it looks like you have prostate cancer.' That was on Friday night. I called my wife, who was here in Florida, and said I'd be right home. I had flown my airplane. [Of course a Marlboro Man like Palmer piloted his own plane.] Picked up my wife and daughter, Amy, and flew to the Mayo Clinic on Sunday. I had a major physical on Monday, a prostate exam by my surgeon on Tuesday, and on Wednesday morning he operated on me. I spent Thursday in the hospital, and on Friday I flew back to Florida."

Palmer went public with his cancer. He went at it with ferocity, the same way he went at his opponents on the golf course. The Eisenhower Medical Center in Rancho Mirage, California, now includes the Arnold Palmer Prostate Center. He has done PSAs about PSA. If you ask him about cancer, he dives in with both cleats.

I ask Arnie if he is aware of the ongoing dialectic about whether men should get PSA screening. "I am," he says, "and I think it's bullshit! In the hospital room next to me at the Mayo Clinic was a 29-year-old minister. He was having the same procedure as I had. So don't tell me that this is an old man's disease. [It's not impossible that a 29-year-old man had prostate cancer but it would be extremely rare.]

"If I hadn't had those PSAs, I wouldn't have had any idea what was going on inside my body. We were constantly on the watch, and it turned out it was good that we were. I got it done quickly. For whatever it's worth, I'm still here." And he taps the table.

I ask Arnie if he still gets PSA tests and DREs.

"DREs? Is that where they go up your ass?" he asks. "Yup, still get them, too."

Some perspective on the Palmer visit is necessary. Celebrities who become spokespersons for causes have a lot of power. They can do good and they can do bad. I have no idea if Palmer's coming forward to speak about prostate cancer has saved a single life or caused a single man to undergo what some would call a needless procedure. But I admire him for speaking up.

Also, chronicling the stories of celebrities who die of a certain disease does not make that disease more important than any other potentially fatal disease or more important than any other cancer. In Chapter 15 we will hear from "regular" people who have had prostate cancer. But the reason that we look at celebrities and disease so often is that their symptoms, treatment, and recovery are so public. You can learn from them, and that is the value. With a little Googling, for example, I stumbled upon the entire postsurgery lab report for actor Dennis Hopper, who died of prostate cancer in 2010.

As for Arnie's treatment, well, his getting three biopsies before any cancer was found is precisely what opponents of PSA testing say should not be done, particularly since he was 68 at the time. They say don't keep looking and looking and biopsying and biopsying otherwise healthy men until something is found.

But, look, this is Arnold Palmer. His proactive approach—get diagnosis on Friday, get in your airplane on Saturday, get the damn thing taken out on Wednesday—was a function of his aggressive personality. Watchful waiting was mentioned as an option, he says, but he is not a watchful-waiting kind of guy any more than he was a guy willing to pass up a challenging shot on the golf course. He made his choice and he has complete peace of mind because of it.

Palmer now looks at cancer the way he once looked at worthy opponents. It's the disease counterpart of Jack Nicklaus, except that Palmer hates cancer and he does not hate Jack. Nearly three years after his prostate was removed, Palmer's wife, Winnie, died of cancer.

"It was peritoneal carcinoma," he says, not even pausing to get out the phrase. "The cancer was between her stomach and the ovaries. It was undetectable. It was a terrible thing.

"And [daughter] Amy had breast cancer. She had 27 positive nodes. [Again, the specific number comes to him easily.] Her doctor, all the doctors, were very skeptical about her chances. Well, she got treatment and she's fine. Four children. Six grandchildren. She was just here visiting me."

Palmer recognized early, he says, that he was a lung cancer candidate.

"As soon as the Surgeon General came out with his recommendation, I stopped," he said. "Okay, that's not quite true. I went off and on with it. Smoked for six months, didn't smoke for six months. But finally it got to me. I didn't want lung cancer. So in 1971 I quit for good. Never touched another one, never will."

IN 1991, SIX YEARS BEFORE PALMER was diagnosed with prostate cancer and five years before Senator Robert Dole of Kansas opposed Bill Clinton for president, Dole got his diagnosis. He was upfront about having the disease before Palmer was, but he is remembered more for what he said about a postsurgical remedy for erectile dysfunction.

Senator Dole talks to me via phone from his Washington, DC, office.

"I took 30 days or more trying to decide what to do after I got my diagnosis. Elizabeth [his wife, who served as both secretary of transportation and secretary of labor in the 1980s] and I talked it over very carefully. I went to the doctors at Walter Reed. They're not making $1,000 an operation, and they didn't have a dog in this fight, so I listened to them. They told me about watchful waiting, but they thought I should get the operation. And so I did. Their big reason was this: With cancer, you never know. You never know."

Senator Dole sounds as irascible as ever. While we talk, I can't help but think about the spot-on impression Norm MacDonald did of him on *Saturday Night Live*. It was parodistic, sure, but it was also respectful and somehow warm.

Dole's feelings today about his operation, however, are 180 degrees removed from Palmer's.

"I think sometimes what the doctors tell you, as far as incontinence and erectile dysfunction are concerned, they are way too optimistic," Dole says. "They tell you, the way I remember it, 'Oh, you're going to be as good as new, maybe 90 percent on erectile dysfunction and no incontinence.' Well, I don't think that's true.

"From the stuff I've learned since the operation, you will die with it, not from it. So if I had to do it all over again, I would choose the watchful-waiting philosophy. I used to travel around and encourage men to get their PSA taken, but I wondered later if I was maybe giving them bad advice.

"But I will say this. More than once I was stopped at some function or another and someone said to me, 'Thank you for talking about prostate cancer. You saved my life.' So maybe what I did was okay."

Dole's real legacy as a prostate cancer survivor is his Viagra commercials. His willingness to talk about ED got him so much attention and cultural currency that he later had some fun with it in a memorable Pepsi ad that ran during the Super Bowl. It shows him walking along the beach. "It helps me feel youthful and vigorous and most importantly vital again," says Dole in the spot. "What is this amazing product? My faithful little blue friend, an ice-cold Pepsi-Cola."

Dole and his wife were both public figures when he talked about ED, so it took guts to do that, even if he sometimes got paid for it. I ask him if any staff members worried that he would damage his virile image and thus his political standing.

"Heck, no," says Dole. "What I heard mostly from people around me was 'Where can I get the stuff?' "

FRANK ZAPPA DIED IN DECEMBER 1993. His last brief interview is available on YouTube. It furnishes a haunting image of the ravages of prostate cancer. His voice is weak, his hair and beard have gone gray, his complexion is yellow, he looks a hundred years old. Only a few months before that he had been interviewed on the *Today* show, a clip you can find on YouTube. He didn't look great and not at all like the frazzled maniac I had seen on stage in 1970 when he fronted the Mothers of Invention, but he didn't look like he was dying either. When he started to go, he went fast. Zappa had been diagnosed with prostate cancer in 1990 but figured he had been living with the disease for a number of years before that.

"Is there anything you want to say about prostate cancer?" the interviewer asks him.

"Well, it's worthwhile being examined," Zappa says. "On the other hand, over a period of years I had had urinary problems and they didn't find it. That's why it came as such a shock to me when they told me I had it. You can imagine how irate a person might be when he finds out, yes, you have cancer, but we can't operate on it."

Zappa was not exactly a health nut—he puffs away on a cigarette as the *Today* correspondent asks him questions about cancer, and it's within the realm of possibility that he took a few drugs during his day. "To me, a cigarette is food," he tells the interviewer. "Tobacco is my favorite vegetable."

Johnny Ramone, guitarist for the seminal four-chord punk band, was three years older than Zappa when he died of prostate cancer at age 55 in September 2004. Ramone, whose real name was

John Cummings—the Ramones took their last name in honor of Paul McCartney, who used to check into hotels under the alias of "Paul Ramon"—had gotten his diagnosis four years earlier and had received doses of chemotherapy.

Johnny didn't talk much about prostate cancer and died quietly, two years after the group he cofounded was inducted into the Rock and Roll Hall of Fame. The Ramones were indeed a star-crossed bunch of musicians. Joey (born Jeff Hyman) died of lymphatic cancer in 2001. Dee Dee (Douglas Colvin) died of a drug overdose in 2002. Johnny, a political conservative who thanked George W. Bush at the hall of fame induction ceremony, was known for taking care of himself, staying away from drugs, drinking only in moderation, and working out.

Speaking of drugs, Timothy Leary, the Harvard professor who proselytized for LSD, died of prostate cancer in 1996 at age 75. He had been diagnosed just one year earlier.

Dan Fogelberg, a musician who went at his craft more quietly than Zappa and Johnny—more quietly than Leary, too—died of prostate cancer in 2007, three years after he was diagnosed. Through the efforts of his widow, proceeds from some of his songs have gone to prostate cancer research.

Prostate cancer killed three celebrated poets, one who won the Nobel Prize in Literature and two who perhaps should have. The Nobel winner was Chile's Pablo Neruda, who died in 1973 at age 69. The other two were Robert Frost, who had a radical prostatectomy in 1962 when he was in his 80s and died shortly afterward, and Langston Hughes, who died in 1967 at age 65. Hughes's death was officially declared as being the result of complications from abdominal surgery related to prostate cancer.

A Nobel winner in two other fields, Chemistry and Peace, Linus Pauling, died of prostate cancer in 1994, three years after he got his diagnosis and after he had received radiation therapy. He was 93.

Bill Bixby, a gentle man who played Dr. David Banner on the television version of *The Incredible Hulk* from 1978 to 1982, died in 1993 at age 59, two years after receiving his diagnosis. Bixby's case is worth a look because it touches on so many aspects of the disease. In January of 1991 he was crippled by a sudden pain in his hip. He visited his proctologist, who performed a digital rectal exam and found an alarmingly large growth. I have no idea if Bixby had gotten PSAs—this was right around the time, remember, that they were becoming SOP—but he said that he had gotten digital rectals on a regular basis. A biopsy, a CAT scan, and a bone scan confirmed a diagnosis of advanced prostate cancer.

Before his radical prostatectomy, Bixby deposited sperm in a Los Angeles sperm bank "just in case Laura [his wife] wanted to have my child, should I die," he told *People* in a March 1993 story. That became a moot point when his wife filed for divorce in the middle of his ordeal.

He felt okay for a while, but the cancer returned and Bixby was told that it had spread to his spine. He continued working but then began taking painkillers. At the UCLA Medical Center he began an eight-week treatment with an experimental drug called suramin, which researchers hoped would halt the spread of the cancer. He was confident. "I want Congress to not build one fighter plane," he said in that 1993 story, "and instead use the money to research suramin."

Eight months after that story, which was somehow full of both dread and hope—*People* knows how to do that—Bixby died.

The two decades since his death give us some perspective. Prostate cancer is in most cases a slow-spreading disease, slower than most cancers. But not always. If we believe Bixby, he had regular visits to his proctologist yet progressed to advanced prostate cancer between six-month exams. It happens.

His deposit in a sperm bank is typical of men who are facing a prostatectomy but still might want to father a child. You will have no sperm after the procedure.

Bixby put some hope behind an experimental drug, which is absolutely understandable. If I were in Bixby's shoes, I would've said, "Bring it on," too. And there was, indeed, hope for suramin. A 1997 entry on the Johns Hopkins urological Web site talks about it in a measured, optimistic tone. But now it is all but forgotten as a possible cure for prostate cancer (though it is being discussed as a treatment for autism). There are always experimental drugs and much hope comes along with them, but at this point there are no drugs to cure any kind of cancer.

Many other celebrities have died, too, and this is by no means a complete list: Merv Griffin, Don Ameche, Hume Cronyn, Hopper, producer Joseph Papp, Earl Woods (father of Tiger), former Canadian prime minister Pierre Trudeau, Bud Abbott (of Abbott and Costello), and Glenn Davis, the 1946 Heisman Trophy winner, to name a few.

At the same time, millions of men have survived prostate cancer, one of the earliest known being Sir Laurence Olivier, who was diagnosed in 1967 and was cured with radiation treatment. (He died of renal failure in 1989.) Other relatively early prostate cancer survivors include—and this is by chronology, not talent—Jerry Lewis (prostatectomy in 1992); Robert Goulet (prostatectomy in 1993); and Harry Belafonte (cancer diagnosed in 1996 and he started with radiation and eventually had surgery after which he became a significant spokesman for prostate cancer awareness).

The clusters of contemporary survivors are fascinating. There are Bonds—Sean Connery and Roger Moore. There are musicians who rock (Springsteen's drummer Max Weinberg) and musicians who jam (Grateful Dead bassist Phil Lesh). There are Democrats (Secretary of State John Kerry) and Republicans (Rudy Giuliani) and at least one politician who is sui generis (Marion Barry). There are generals (Colin Powell) and Navy drill instructors (Louis Gossett Jr.; okay, he was acting). There are coaches from all sports (Joe Torre, baseball; Marv Levy, football; Phil Jackson and George Karl, basketball). There are billionaire media tycoons (Rupert Murdoch) and grizzled bosses (Ed Asner; okay, he was acting, too). There are guys you'd love to see chatting at a cocktail party—evangelist Pat Robertson and Nation of Islam leader Louis Farrakhan, and two guys you might need to referee that conversation, Nelson Mandela and Bishop Desmond Tutu. And there's a guy who could get anyone to that party on time—NASCAR legend Richard Petty.

Perhaps the two most famous ongoing survivors are Warren Buffett and Robert DeNiro. They handled their diagnoses in very different ways. Buffett went public, telling the tale that his cancer was discovered in the classic manner—his PSA jumped, and, as Buffett said, "a biopsy seemed warranted." He also decided that intervention was warranted, and he chose radiation, the most logical course of action for a man in his 80s. In September 2012, he told an Omaha newspaper (which he happens to own), "It's a great day for me. Today I had my 44th and last day of radiation." At this writing, Buffett was doing fine.

DeNiro, whose father died of prostate cancer at age 71, got a diagnosis of early-stage prostate cancer in 2003 but did not reveal his choice of intervention, if any. That is not surprising since the man reviles attention. I once sat across from DeNiro on a flight from Newark to Los Angeles. (I had upgraded on points, but I assume he had the cash to book first class from the beginning.) Anyway, DeNiro came on the plane looking a little haggard. He grabbed a pillow, told the flight attendant he did not want to be disturbed—not for water, not for lunch, not for a pilot's droning rumination on the beauty of the Badlands—and curled himself into a ball in the window seat and went to sleep. He never stirred until we alighted in LA.

CHAPTER 15

... In which the author presents personal prostate stories, ones with both positive and negative outcomes, that may provide guidance

Jeff Jarvis

AGE AT DIAGNOSIS: 55

PSA LEVEL: Unknown, but relatively low

GLEASON SCORE AND BIOPSY REPORT: 3 + 3; 5 percent involvement in one core

DECISION: Robotic prostatectomy

OUTCOME: Mixed

Jeff is a well-known blogger on the subject of Internet rights, and he wrote a seminal book on that subject called *Public Parts*, in which he argues for "publicness," i.e., more openness and less fear of revelation.

Not surprisingly, he has written candidly about his prostate cancer on his blog, the link for which is in this book's Sources and Resources section (page 201). Here is Jeff's story.

"After my biopsy, I asked, 'Is this like Amelia Earhart trying to find the island? One degree off and you wouldn't have found the cancer?' Well, that's possible.

"But once I found out I had cancer, whatever the level of it, there was no doubt what I was going to do. I was already a hypochondriac. I have two kids, and you hear 'cancer,' and the way I see it you get it out. If science knew the difference between fast growing and slow growing, maybe my decision would be different. But they don't.

"Before I did anything, I talked to David Agus, a doctor who wrote *The End of Illness*. His advice was to get treated.

"At about the time I was diagnosed, Rudy Giuliani was getting radiation seeding. I thought, 'I'll have that, please.' But I was going to Sloan-Kettering for my treatment, and they told me about how difficult it might be [to do it] if a prostatectomy was needed after radiation. So I said, 'I want the robotic method.'

"As far as urinary continence goes, I had a drip there, a drab there, but nothing serious. You do your exercises and that goes away.

"But sexually? I'm dead as a doornail down there. I took Viagra prophylactically. I have a heart condition, so I was nervous about taking anything else. Yes, I can stimulate myself—you don't have to worry about having tissues anymore because of the dry orgasm—but I can't have intercourse.

"I tried a few pumps. I actually went into a porn store for one and it's true that you get what you pay for. Then I got a prescription for one—shameful how they gouge desperate people. In short, it's worse than inefficient. It distorts the body part and does little else.

"How do I feel about my decision? Well, once in a while I'll say to myself, 'Did I get screwed?' Obviously, I mean that metaphorically because literally, it's not happening. And then I feel bad for myself.

"On the other hand, I'm still grateful I did it. My grandfather died of prostate cancer. I've known people who have died of prostate cancer. I didn't want to be one of them.

"And I am angry about the USPSTF recommendation against PSA testing. I take the Internet attitude on this. More information is better. You have a right to have information about your body. The problem is not information; the problem is what to do with the information.

"When you make judgments across a statistical pool, as the USPSTF did, okay, you reach some conclusions. But I'm not a pool. I'm one person. And I'm not going to play the odds.

"I think it's vital that men know about prostate cancer and PSAs and all other information. Women did an incredible job of getting out the message about breast cancer and it saved lives. There was a time when you couldn't even use 'breast' on the Internet. At first AOL put it on their list of dirty words and so people couldn't even research the subject of 'breast cancer.'

"'Penis' is the same way today. And then to have a panel come out and say you shouldn't get tested? You shouldn't have information about yourself? That's crazy.

"Okay, if I were 82-year-old Warren Buffett, maybe then I'd say screw it. But I wasn't ready to screw it."

TAKEAWAY: Jeff's situation was similar to mine. Active-surveillance advocates would say we were good candidates for it, but we thought about our families and ourselves. We didn't want to live with cancer. His outcome—good on incontinence, not so good on potency—is not unusual. I'm doing better than Jeff.

His early flirtation with radiation seeding was influenced by Giuliani. That is typical. Our society frequently learns about disease from celebrities. But Jeff thought about it and concluded that he wanted to go in a different direction.

As for his experience with pumps, well, I haven't used one, and I'm still waiting for someone to wholly endorse them. And I sure as hell wouldn't buy one in a porn store.

Bob Snyder

AGE AT DIAGNOSIS: 66

PSA LEVEL: About 5

GLEASON SCORE AND BIOPSY REPORT: 3 + 3;
15 percent involvement in one core

DECISION: Active surveillance

OUTCOME: So far, so good

Bob was one of the people who contacted me after my first column about choosing active surveillance. I was happy to hear from him since most people I talked to had elected some form of intervention. Here is Bob's story.

"After going through my annual physical with my internist, I was referred to a local urologist for follow-up because of a growth on my prostate that he had felt during palpation. My urologist indicated that I should have a PSA test and then a biopsy. The results indicated that the growth on my prostate was benign, but that 15 percent of one of the other biopsy samples indicated prostate cancer.

"My urologist put all the results of tests and other information through Sloan-Kettering's Web-based prostate cancer [outcome-prediction tool], and this indicated that intervention via radiation or surgery would only increase my 'living to old age' by 2 percent. The result said [my odds of long-term survival were] 97 percent if we did active surveillance versus 99 percent if I would select some type of intervention.

"Your article in the paper that indicated you have chosen surgery rather than active surveillance made me think about getting another opinion and possibly following your lead to Hopkins. But the bottom line is that I have decided not to get any more opinions outside of my internist and my urologist. My PSA tests have been about the same number for the past 18 months and my next biopsy is due in May 2013. I will continue to see my urologist for my six-month follow-ups, have my PSA checked every six months, and have a biopsy every two years, or sooner, if it's indicated.

"Although I chose active surveillance, I think all men over a certain age should allow themselves the time to be checked for prostate cancer so they will have treatment choices before it is too late to have these choices."

TAKEAWAY: Bob made a carefully considered decision and seems comfortable with it. He did his research and explored his options. He thought about what he was doing. And if he gets a higher PSA reading in the future, he can change his decision. The link to the Sloan-Kettering Web page he mentioned is in Sources and Resources (page 203).

Jim Mikitka

AGE AT DIAGNOSIS: 48

PSA LEVEL: 2.4

GLEASON SCORE AND BIOPSY REPORT:
Unknown; minor core involvement and localized

DECISION: Robotic prostatectomy

OUTCOME: Good

Jim was one of the most enthusiastic responders to my prostate columns. He had done extensive research on robotic surgery and was gung ho about how well it had worked for him. But he also said this: "Everyone's body is different, and none of the research out there is exact. You have to make the best decision for yourself and not look back." Here is Jim's story.

"I had been followed for prostate cancer starting at age 40 because my father and his five brothers were all diagnosed with the disease at some point in their life. My dad didn't believe in going to doctors, and when he was diagnosed at 70, the prostate cancer had spread outside of his gland and into his bones. They treated him for six years with chemo and hormone treatments, but were finally unable to control his disease. The last seven years of his life were not of high quality and were a difficult time for all of us.

"I'll never forget what his oncologist told my brother and I when my father was diagnosed in the hospital: 'The best way to control cancer is to diagnose it as early as possible and remove it from your body.' That's when she told my brother and I to start screening at 40.

"At age 48, my PSA came back at 2.4, still well below what they consider normal, but the trend over time had shown an increase from the previous year. They repeated the test with the same result, and, although the urologist didn't feel anything in the digital rectal exam, he recommended a biopsy. The results came back positive and confined to one area of the prostate. He was confident it had been caught early and was still contained, and he recommended the traditional open method of surgery to remove it.

"My wife and I did a ton of research and I ended up with two other opinions from doctors trained in robotic surgery. They both agreed I should get it out. I had surgery on December 3, 2008, and walked out of the hospital the next day feeling fine.

"My PSA tests since have all come back negative. I've had little to no incontinence since the surgery, and amazingly, the sexual function has also returned."

TAKEAWAY: Jim's story is notable for a couple reasons, the first being the heredity angle. A 2002 review study published in the *Journal of Urology* provides a detailed look at that connection. There are lots of parsings in the study, but here's an example: A man with one brother who was diagnosed with prostate cancer before the age of 60 is three times more likely to develop prostate cancer than a man with no family history of it. And Jim had extensive prostate cancer in his genes.

The second interesting part of Jim's account is his low PSA reading. Remember that low PSAs sometimes disguise cancer just as high PSAs frequently indicate BPH and not cancer.

Also, there's a high probability that the full return of Jim's sexual function had a lot to do with his relatively young age when he was treated. As Dr. Patrick Walsh explains in his *Guide to Surviving Prostate Cancer*, men lose nerves as they age. (Not "nerve"—"nerves.") Dr. Walsh says that by age 60 the average male has throughout his body only about 60 percent of the nerves he was born with. Combine that with nerve loss from surgery and the difficulty with erection becomes clearer. At 48, Jim had a better chance than, say, a 60-year-old of getting an erection, and a much, much better chance than a 70-year-old, up to 75 percent of whom are impotent after surgery.

That is another reason that the decision for intervention is a befuddling matter for younger men: Risking loss of potency is a more serious matter, but there's also a better chance that post-intervention potency will return.

Kevin Snyder

AGE AT DIAGNOSIS: 58

PSA LEVEL: Between 5 and 6

GLEASON SCORE AND BIOPSY REPORT: 3 + 3; involvement in five cores

DECISION: Robotic prostatectomy

OUTCOME: Pretty good

Kevin was one of the men who stayed in touch after reading my columns in the *Morning Call.* Here is his story.

"My maternal grandfather was diagnosed with prostate cancer in his mid- to late 70s. He had radiation treatment and died 10 years later from causes unrelated to prostate cancer. I have an uncle who had radiation treatment for prostate cancer when he was in his 60s and is still alive today at 88. So prostate cancer is in my family.

"Like you, I was seriously considering active surveillance, but my urologist was dead set against it. He told me at my age (58), I should consider having the surgery.

"So I scheduled a meeting with one of two surgeons who would be doing the surgery. I figured the surgeon was going to echo my urologist's recommendation, but he threw me a curveball and started to give me all of the treatment options, including active surveillance. So now I was a little more confused and had to make some more decisions. But I decided I would have the robotic and so far everything seems to be progressing as well as can be expected.

"My Gleason was only 3 + 3, so I thought I was a low-risk patient. But after the surgery, my doctor informed me that nearly 20 percent of my prostate was cancerous and that I was up against the margin. I'm very happy I did not choose active surveillance.

"I still have leakage and continue to wear a pad, but only one a day to be safe, and it's never saturated. The doctor has me doing the Kegel exercises again. Surgery may stop the incontinence, but the procedure might make it more difficult to empty one's bladder, so there is no perfect solution. I'm getting used to wearing the pads and am no longer embarrassed to buy them. It is what it is.

"All in all, I am happy with my decision. In fact, I am now on a billboard promoting men's health and prostate-related issues that's sponsored by Urology Specialists of the Lehigh Valley. Think of me when you pass the billboard, and I'll think of you."

TAKEAWAY: What I found most interesting about Kevin's story was the dueling opinions—get the surgery; no, consider active surveillance—he got in the same urology office. I have heard that from other men. As we all know by now, there are differing opinions about treatment and doctors do not speak with one voice. But it's extremely discomfiting for a patient to have one doctor be so positive about one thing and then have his colleague come along and muddy the water. Yes, the waters are often muddy from the get-go, but urologists from the same office should at least have a unified message, even if that message is that there are options.

Even though post-prostatectomy patients tend to struggle more with ED than incontinence, Kevin's battle with his urinary function is hardly rare. There are remedies both surgical and prescriptive, but you know how remedies are—they often bring with them their own set of problems.

Bill Moss

AGE AT DIAGNOSIS: 70

PSA LEVEL: 4.8

GLEASON SCORE AND BIOPSY REPORT: 3 + 4; involvement in five cores

DECISION: Robotic prostatectomy

OUTCOME: Life altering

Among the e-mails I received after my second column appeared was one from Anne Moss. She was writing about a robotic procedure that her husband, Bill, a retired engineer, had undergone. She mentioned a regional hospital and a specific surgeon and wrote, "PLEASE PLEASE reconsider your decision to have robotic surgery if it is going to be with this man at this hospital. He is a butcher. My husband had a bad, life-altering experience after robotic surgery."

I exchanged e-mails with Anne, who had worked in hospitals as a technician, and subsequently met with her and Bill on two occasions. Here is Bill's story.

"I was offered all of the options, including radiation and active surveillance," says Bill. "But I was also told I was an excellent candidate for surgery since I was in good shape, so I decided to go that route. Some of the guys I play golf with told me, 'Robotic is nothing. It's a no-brainer. You'll come through it fine.'

"After the procedure, I woke up in excruciating pain. I'll never forget that the patient in the bed next to me had had the same surgery the day before, with a different surgeon, and he was getting dressed to leave. I was in the hospital for seven days, in pain all the while."

Anne picks up the story.

"While Bill was lying there in agony I noticed that his Foley catheter was not filling with urine even though he was getting lots of IV fluid. I alerted the nurse and I could tell she was concerned. His JP drain, though, was full. [Note: The Jackson Pratt drain is used for collecting fluids draining from surgical sites. It is not specific to prostate cancer. My surgeon, Dr. Lee, does not use it. He says that it might be used by inexperienced or less confident surgeons or for more serious procedures.]

"Our surgeon came in and he could tell something wasn't right. But you know what he said? 'You signed a release.' That floored us."

Even after leaving the hospital, Bill had pain that "sent me to my knees." Anne took him to the emergency room on one occasion because the pain was so intense they thought he might be having a heart attack.

"I had the catheter in for six weeks, but even during that time urine was running out," says Bill. "I kept a towel wrapped around my leg all the time. And whenever we saw the surgeon, his response was always, 'This is normal.'"

The catheter came out after six weeks, but the JP drain remained. As did the uncontrollable flow of urine. "It was like he was a baby again," says Anne. "It was very, very difficult." And Bill had been a faithful Kegeler; he had tested off the charts for pelvic muscularity.

The Mosses tried to live a normal life, but it was impossible. "I peed my way through the Philadelphia Flower Show," remembers Bill, and on the way home, he turned to his wife and said, "If I have to live like this, I don't want to live." Anne cried. "That really, really scared me," she says.

They eventually saw a urologist in Philadelphia, who gave Bill an artificial sphincter that is fitted between his anus and testicles to help him urinate and give him more control. Anne and Bill say they are happy with his current urological care, but still don't know exactly what went wrong during the robotic procedure.

Bill was in the operating room for $5\frac{1}{2}$ hours. That is at least $2\frac{1}{2}$ hours longer than normal and a full 4 hours longer than I was in with Dr. Lee.

"When I asked the surgeon about it, he said, 'Oh, I had trouble with the robot,'" says Anne. "A da Vinci representative did go into the OR during the procedure. But when we called the company, they said it was 'privileged information.'

"When I talked to the chief of surgery, he said, 'Oh, no, the doctor didn't have a problem with the machine. He just had a problem with an electric cord.' He also told us that the surgeon had some difficulty because of a previous surgery that Bill had had. But that was on his kidney. That shouldn't affect a prostate procedure."

The Mosses pursued legal action, but could never get anywhere. "The urologist we have now knows that the surgeon did something wrong," says Anne, "but he won't testify against him."

The artificial sphincter, though clearly not in the category of earth's most enjoyable devices, has given Bill decent urinary control. He still wears a small pad and feels squirts when he takes a golf swing, but he says it's bearable. His sexual function is pretty much gone—continuous urine leakage went a long way toward deadening the nerves, never mind the damage that was done during the procedure. He and Anne used to enjoy bike riding, but they don't do that anymore because his device makes sitting on a seat very uncomfortable. Both his urologist and his family physician have him on duloxetine (Cymbalta), which is used to treat depression and anxiety disorder.

"I didn't really think I needed it," says Bill.

"Well, they knew what you went through," I suggest, "and they probably thought, 'Now, there's a guy who must be depressed.'"

Life is better for Bill now. He's back to playing golf and enjoying his family. "I'll always be like this," says Bill. "But, hey, I'm alive."

TAKEAWAY: The USPSTF would use Bill Moss as a poster boy to point out the dangers of surgical intervention. And some would say that at 70, he was too old for surgery and that radiation might've been better. But Bill didn't do anything radically against the book. Even at his age, he was in good shape for surgery. And someone in his family had developed leukemia after radiation, so he was fearful of that procedure. People make decisions like that every day, and they are completely understandable.

The Mosses thought they had the correct man to do surgery. He was chief of urology at the hospital and talked a good game. But it turned out that he had done very few unassisted robotic procedures. A prospective patient should make sure that his surgeon is a veteran.

Without knowing the specifics of the case, the best guess offered by Dr. Lee was that Bill's surgeon botched sewing the bladder to the urethra.

I also asked Dr. Lee if the robot routinely fails during surgery. "That has happened to me twice," he said. "I am pretty confident that I know how to fix it. But we are fortunate that we have two robots, and we wheeled the other one in to complete the procedures.

"The problem is, if the robot goes down and you don't have another one, time passes. Now you have to complete the procedure by the open method or by using laparoscopic instruments. And not everyone is trained in those methods. That can be very dangerous."

So if you're having a robotic procedure and you're the kind of person who believes in worst-case outcomes, find out if your surgeon is skilled enough to perform the operation using another method. I confess to not having thought about that until I heard Bill's story. It turns out that Dr. Lee, like many other robotic specialists, was trained in all methods, but I'm glad I didn't have to find that out.

In Sources and Resources at the end of this book, you will find my e-mail address. You may contact me to find out the identity of Bill's surgeon. I will also provide you with contact information for the Mosses. They would love to hear from you and could use your support.

Robert Keiber

AGE AT DIAGNOSIS: 51

PSA LEVEL: 5.4

GLEASON SCORE AND BIOPSY REPORT: 3 + 3 and 3 + 4; involvement in two cores

DECISION: Open prostatectomy

OUTCOME: Mixed, but generally pleased

The Keibers were among the first to respond to my columns about prostate cancer, partly because Bob's wife, Sandy, is an operating room nurse. I found their story interesting because it started to unfold 15 years ago, when the world of prostate cancer awareness was different than it is now. Here is Bob's story.

"I made Bob go for a physical in 1998," says Sandy. "He had started getting up a lot to urinate and I noticed changes in intercourse. It was just . . . inconsistent. He was 47 then. It was too young for that to be happening.

"I told the doctor we wanted a PSA and he said, 'Are you kidding? He's not 50, so he doesn't need it.' But I insisted. It wasn't talked about much back then. The only reason I knew anything about the prostate was because I was an OR nurse. It was only after his physical that I found out that Bob's father had died of prostate cancer."

Bob's reading came back at 3.5. Four years later, he went back for another physical. The result was 5.4, and the bells went off. The Keibers decided immediately that they would choose intervention.

"The robot was experimental at that time, so that really wasn't an option," says Robert. "I met with a surgeon and a radiologist, but I only knew about active surveillance because I read extensively. [Bob is a retired high school history teacher.] I decided on surgery because I had heard that with radiation there was no going back in. I had the operation three weeks after 9/11. The fact that that tragedy went on certainly gave me strength to go through this."

As is so often the case, Robert's cancer was nearer the capsule than anticipated. He had his catheter in for three weeks, which was more the norm a decade ago. After his catheter was extracted, he stood up and urinated all over the floor. "I still remember I turned to my wife and said, 'Oh, my God,'" says Robert. "It was so mortifying."

Robert had a rough recovery and things still aren't perfect. He still wears a pad—a sudden cough or laugh will produce a few squirts—and medication-aided intercourse is "not quite the same as it used to be," says Sandy. It took Robert 2½ years to get to the point where he could have an erection.

But his PSAs have been near zero, he doesn't have regrets, and the couple's feelings about the USPSTF recommendation are clear: "I was appalled by it," says Sandy. "When I consider the family history, the age when he got it, and the PSA number, I think he'd be dead if he hadn't gotten the test a second time."

The Keibers were high school sweethearts—"Same class, same friends, just had our 45th class reunion," says Sandy—and they have leaned on each other throughout the ordeal.

"A couple we're close to went through the same thing we did," says Sandy. "The man had always lived and died by his sexuality, but now we don't even talk about it. And talking about it helps a lot."

TAKEAWAY: Sandy's conviction that her husband would be dead if not for a PSA test cannot, of course, be proven. He did have a family history of prostate cancer and his PSA did rise from 3.5 to 5.4 in four years, a significant velocity. There is a reasonable argument that because of the family history he should've been tested when he was 40, and there is a more than reasonable argument that a 3.5 reading at age 47 should be taken more seriously than the same reading at age 67.

"Our family physician either missed or did not recognize that number as high for Bob's age," says Sandy. "At that time, only PSA readings over 4 were highlighted on the computer readouts. Diagnoses would be better if the computer made age-related adjustments."

Gene Wieder

AGE AT DIAGNOSIS: 68

PSA LEVEL: 3.8

GLEASON SCORE AND BIOPSY REPORT: 4 + 4; confined to one core

DECISION: Radiation

OUTCOME: So far, so good

After my articles were published, I found myself in the disconcerting position of dispensing advice. When Gene first contacted me, he wrote, "I have chosen to start radiation treatments but am reconsidering my treatment decision. So please help me convince myself that I made the right choice."

I wrote Gene back with my predictable reply—that I am not a doctor—but did mention that I had heard from several men who had done quite well with radiation. Here is Gene's story.

"My Gleason score was 4 + 4. My urologist considered that high and that's why he recommended radiation. He said that even if I'd chosen surgery he would've still recommended follow-up radiation in case the areas around the prostate were cancerous. I don't recall him mentioning my age (68 at the time) as being a factor in the treatment decision.

"My nine-week course of radiation went well and my follow-up PSA was 0.1. I have no incontinence issues. The urologist has me on Trelstar [triptorelan], a treatment received via injection. It blocks testosterone production. But it has reduced my sexual function to zero and causes me to experience an occasional hot flash. It has also taken a few yards off my drives, but doesn't seem to affect my putting one way or the other. In other words, I still miss too many."

TAKEAWAY: Gene was in what Dr. Walsh calls "the gray area of treatment." His Gleason 8 was a significant reading, but his PSA and his cancer staging (T1c and not T2c or T3) suggested that he did not have high-risk disease. He could've had surgery since he was in otherwise good health, but his age (creeping up on 70) and that troublesome Gleason may have convinced his doctor that radiation was best.

When you're in "the gray zone," Dr. Walsh recommends that you ponder the worst-case scenario for each option five years down the road.

If you choose surgery, try to imagine what life would be like if you were impotent and incontinent, for they are its worst-case outcomes. Although prostate removal doesn't always get rid of all the cancer, it does most of the time.

If you choose radiation, try to imagine what life would be like if your PSA began to rise, which happens much more often with radiation and would require additional radiation or hormone treatments. That's why Gene's doctor already has him on Trelstar.

One thing to remember is that even urologists and surgeons who used to be wary of radiation now say that it is an excellent and indispensable modality in many cases. But Gene's story illustrates the blessed curse of prostate cancer: Having multiple options seems preferable to having just one. But it also makes your decision more difficult.

Jack Littley

AGE AT DIAGNOSIS: 60

PSA LEVEL: About 1

GLEASON SCORE AND BIOPSY REPORT: 3 + 4;
involvement in one core

DECISION: Cryotherapy

OUTCOME: Mixed

When I was a freshman at Oakcrest High School in southern New Jersey, I attended my first scholastic wrestling match. Jack Littley, a junior and already an established jock at our school, was a 136-pounder who went up to 148 to take on a star from Atlantic City High School. Jack crushed him. The memory stayed with me. The captain of both the football and wrestling squads, Jack was one of the toughest competitors I've ever known.

Jack married one of my oldest friends, Sharon Suprun. It was from Sharon that I learned about Jack's battle with prostate cancer that, like so many others, shouldn't have been as bad as it was. Here is the account from Jack, who is the chief performance officer for a technology firm in Virginia.

"My younger brother had prostate cancer, so I figured I had better get checked. My PSA was low, but the doctor thought I should still have a biopsy because of the family history. My insurance company wouldn't even pay for the biopsy because of that PSA number. But, sure enough, it came up positive for prostate cancer.

"You know how it is, right? You start to feel a time bomb in there. I felt like I didn't have time to think about it, but I really did. Unfortunately, I did all my research after the fact, not before.

"My brother had had radiation in Philadelphia, but I didn't want to go up there. I was thinking about robotic surgery, but then there was some publicity about a real bad incident when somebody almost bled to death during robotic [which usually reduces blood loss], so I ruled that out. Then I checked with my minister, who had had radiation seeds [brachytherapy], but he had a problem with anal leakage.

"My urologist was an older guy, but I trusted him—sort of—and he started talking to Sharon and I about cryotherapy. Showed us a couple of films, went through the positives—didn't hurt the nerves, gets rid of the cancer, on and on—and I said, 'Okay, let's just get this over with.' So I had the procedure. It was less than a month from the time I had been diagnosed.

"The post-procedure time was a lot more difficult than I had been led to believe. My testicles were the size of grapefruits. I always wanted to have big balls, but not like that. The urologist told me, 'Go home and squeeze the fluid out of them.' Really? That went on for about six weeks, but they finally came down to regular size.

"After that I couldn't get an erection. Viagra and the other things didn't work, so I started giving myself a shot directly into the penis. The needle goes all the way through, but, oddly, it doesn't hurt. It worked a couple of times, didn't work other times, and eventually it became . . . I guess the word for it is 'demoralizing.'

"So the urologist gave me a pump. It worked in his office, but then I bought one and it didn't work. Eventually, that became demoralizing, too. I am now on Cialis [tadalafil] for daily use and it's not working very well. One thing you think about before the procedure is 'Well, if something happens with ED, I'm 60 and we're not having sex as often as we used to, so how much am I going to miss it?' Well, that is true. You don't have it as often. But you do miss it.

"And when I manage to have an orgasm I sometimes feel a burning sensation. It feels like it's in the rectum, but it's probably backwash into the bladder. I also have an irritation in the perineum [the area between the testicles and the anus]. Some itching and pain when I exercise. But all the scopes and everything always come up negative, so it must just be some kind of reaction to the procedure.

"All in all, it's been a pretty negative experience, a lot more negative than it should've been. But my PSAs are negligible, I don't have cancer, and I'm alive."

TAKEAWAY: As is so often the case, both sides of the PSA debate can claim Jack.

One side: He shouldn't have been biopsied in the first place and then he rushed into getting harmful treatment.

The other side: He never would've discovered his cancer had an alert physician not insisted upon his getting a biopsy because of the family history. And he had cancer despite the fact that his PSA was extremely low.

Jack, who has an engineering degree from Rutgers University, is a smart guy. He was smart in the classroom and smart on the athletic field. But like thousands of others, he felt pressured to do something after he got his cancer diagnosis. He heard bad things about two procedures, so he went with cryotherapy without doing enough research on it, or, more to the point, enough research on the doctor who was doing it.

Jack's story should not be considered a blanket indictment of cryo. I can only tell you that on my interview scale it did not come off well because of the high possibility of side effects. But had Jack put himself in Dr. Aaron Katz's hands, perhaps it would've turned out differently.

The shot to the penis that Jack describes is not an uncommon remedy. The medication dilates the arteries and allows blood to flow in. Urologicalcare.com (which does not appear to be in bed with the companies that manufacture the medication or the injection kit) reports that 80 percent of men achieved erections in clinical trials. Well, maybe that's accurate, and Jack did say it worked for a while. But as Jack found with the pump, the success didn't last, and it seemed more trouble than it was worth.

But his life is not over. He continues to share good times with Sharon, and he's picked up some wisdom along the way.

"The trouble is that most doctors get locked in on a solution," says Jack. "What we really need in medicine is an adjudicator, someone who's in the field but not a practitioner and can say, 'Okay, here are your options, and here's what is probably best for you.' Instead, I got very biased opinions, sort of like mutual fund salesmen pushing me in the direction of their own funds."

Richard Grammes

AGE AT DIAGNOSIS: 66

PSA LEVEL: 11.5

GLEASON SCORE AND BIOPSY REPORT: 6 + 7; involvement in 11 of 12 cores

DECISION: Open prostatectomy and subsequent radiation due to rising PSA

OUTCOME: Mixed

The memory of his father's lost battle with prostate cancer was seared into Richard Grammes's brain. Here is his story.

"The radiation treatment my father had was nothing like it is now. It never helped him. He was always sick and always in pain. He had severe bleeding and eventually lost his bladder. He was a big man who dwindled to under 100 pounds. My father was in such agony that he shot himself with a pistol. It was really difficult for my whole family and especially for me because we were very close."

Despite that history, Richard did not get his own PSA level checked until he was 66. "I didn't have any urinary symptoms, no problems at all related to my prostate," says Richard. "So I was under the assumption everything was fine." But by the time he got it checked, his reading was 11.5 and a biopsy revealed significant involvement. He chose to have an open prostatectomy with the urologist who was treating him.

Richard had some incontinence and wore pads for a few months, but eventually got it under control. "But from then on, I was unable to perform in the bedroom," he says. "Every time I would get close to something happening, I would have leakage and that would ruin it. In retrospect, the one thing I regret was that I didn't hear more about the sexual part. If I had, I would've taken my wife on a trip or something."

Still, Richard was initially satisfied with his outcome, especially when his first postsurgical PSA came back at 0.04. But then it started to rise with each subsequent test. "It really left me confused," he says. "I thought, *That isn't supposed to happen*. Then I began to do the research and found that, yes, it does happen."

When his PSA reached 0.17, his urologist decided that he should get radiation. At this writing, he is in the middle of a 39-treatment regimen.

"I'm fine with the radiation, but it's not without stress," says Richard. "They have to get three people involved in your treatment. In my case, it's three young ladies, all of whom are attractive."

"Perhaps if your erectile function is ever to return," I suggest, "it will be during your treatment."

"That would be great," he says. "I wonder what my doctor would do in that case. Probably raise a flag."

TAKEAWAY: Richard's story again highlights the connection between prostate cancer and heredity. He should've been tested earlier because of his father's history.

And we get from him another comment about his doctors' not providing enough pre-intervention information about side effects. As Richard notes, it would've been nice if he and his wife had been able to enjoy a memorable sexual engagement before the procedure. In fact, that recommendation should be de rigueur. Surgeons must be frank enough to say, "Sex may never be the same after your treatment."

The rising PSA level after surgery is not unusual, particularly in cases like Richard's where the cancer was significant. And the decision to follow up with radiation is standard operating procedure. Although, as I said before, I am not a doctor, it seems as if repeating PSAs to monitor such situations is extremely important.

Here is a link to an American Cancer Society forum in which men who are facing Richard's dilemma talk about it: http://csn.cancer.org/node/148932.

Bob Fink

AGE AT DIAGNOSIS: 63

PSA LEVEL: 4.2

GLEASON SCORE AND BIOPSY REPORT: 3 + 4; involvement in two cores and metastasis

DECISION: Radiation

OUTCOME: Problematic

I was 12 when Bob, a lifelong friend, threw me the first curveball I ever saw. The pitch was coming directly toward me so I jumped out of the way, then watched with amazement as it swooped over the plate. Fifty years later I can still see his diabolical grin out on the mound.

Because of the timing of his call, I thought Bob was joking when he told me that he had prostate cancer. It came when I was recovering from my surgery and still had the catheter wedged in me.

"You're bullshitting me," I said. "You can't even let me beat you with prostate cancer."

"God's honest," he said. "And guess what? I'm not a candidate for a prostatectomy. The cancer has escaped the prostate wall." Bob let loose a rueful laugh. "With all the other stuff that's happened to me, somebody up there must hate me." Here is Bob's story.

"I was shocked when I got the news about prostate cancer. I had my PSAs done religiously. In fact, my doctor used to joke that the only thing healthy about me was my prostate. The readings had always been around 2.5 or 2.6, and suddenly it went to 4.2. That's when I had the biopsy and got the result.

"The only option I was given was regular radiation or proton beam radiation. That turned out to be no option at all since my insurance denied the proton on the basis that it hasn't been proven any more effective."

Bob's radiation regimen at Penn wasn't easy. I know because I did it with him one morning. He was on the road by 5:15 a.m. five days a week for a 100-mile round trip to Philadelphia. He got his therapy (which was generally performed efficiently), hit the southbound lanes of the Atlantic City Expressway, and was at his desk job (he worked in medical records) by 8:30 a.m. "I never missed one minute of work during those seven weeks," he says. "But I was extremely fatigued. I guess that's not surprising with the combination of getting up early, two hours on the road, the radiation, and the job. And since the radiation ended, I still feel fatigued a lot of the time."

But Bob doesn't necessarily blame the cancer treatment for his fatigue and downticks in libido and sexual performance. He has been on a buffet of other medications, including tamsulosin, the generic form of Flomax, that has brought relative normalcy to his urination. Once a person starts taking a cornucopia of medications, even the most skilled physician has trouble determining what is causing what. But he is definitely not, well, enchanted with the results of his radiation.

"I have had nothing but problems from the radiation," says Bob. "The side effects are getting worse. Two weeks ago I was hemorrhaging so badly my boss sent me home and to my gastro doc where he set up a colonoscopy for me two days later. I had to wear feminine pads to work and everywhere I went prior to that. We were thinking colon cancer. The colonoscopy showed severe radiation burning and damage to the blood vessels. He cauterized as many as he could and said I might have to return for another colonoscopy if the bleeding continues. It's been a week and the bleeding is minor."

All things considered, though, Bob is not complaining. (I can't tell you how many times I heard that from members of the Prostate Cancer Club.)

"Since March of 2010, I've survived a stroke to the left side of my body, had surgery to repair two holes in my heart, suffered a heart attack, and won a battle with cancer," he says. "Yes, life is great! But we're both classified as cancer survivors, right? And that's all we could've hoped for."

TAKEAWAY: The curveballer certainly got thrown a curveball by prostate cancer. Bob had stayed on top of his PSAs and his DREs, yet when cancer was found it was already outside of his prostate. So to the idea that prostate cancer grows slowly we can also add: but not always.

Remember? There are no rules.

Plus, I can almost hear PSA advocate Dr. Catalona suggesting that a biopsy could've been done when Bob's PSA hit 2.6. Perhaps that would've made a difference. Perhaps not.

The refusal of Bob's insurance plan to cover proton beam radiation therapy is common. The issue of the relative effectiveness of proton beam versus intensity-modulated radiation is analogous to that of robotic prostatectomy versus the traditional open method: A brave-new-world treatment comes along. It's better in some respects than the traditional way, but it's also more expensive. At the same time, improvements keep being made to the "old" way, partly because the "new" way is such a worthy competitor. So ... is the new treatment better in the long run?

A study that tracked nearly 28,000 prostate cancer patients determined, according to its lead author, James Yu, MD, a radiation oncologist at Yale, that as far as side effects go, "in the long term, there's really no difference in outcomes between proton radiation and IMRT for men with prostate cancer." At this writing, that seems to be the most complete study available. But it's not necessarily the last word.

Radiation oncologists form a plan for a patient's treatment. For reasons that surpasseth the understanding of this book's author, proton beam may more ideally fit one patient's anatomy than IMRT, just as the reverse might be true. Penn's Dr. John Christodouleas offers this comparison: "Proton beam is a hammer and IMRT is a screwdriver, so what's left to decide is whether a patient's body is more nail or screw."

One person who contacted me about my newspaper columns is a strong advocate for the hammer. "I truly believe that proton beam radiation saved my life," says Larry Christoff, a 60-year-old retired teacher. That is entirely understandable. If you have a successful intervention, that will be your belief. I would not tell anyone that "robotic surgery saved my life" because I don't believe my life was in danger. But I would sure as hell defend it.

As Dr. C. sees it, however, the differences between the two radiological modalities aren't that great. Radiation oncologists, not to mention patients, would of course prefer that insurance plans cover both options, but in most cases, either has a chance of being successful in treating prostate cancer.

Paul Rosen

AGE AT DIAGNOSIS: 67

PSA LEVEL: 7

GLEASON SCORE AND BIOPSY REPORT: 3 + 4; involvement in two cores

DECISION: Radiation

OUTCOME: Complicated by ongoing Ferris wheel of PSA readings

Eight years ago, just before he was to be married, Paul was diagnosed with prostate cancer (via the usual route, an elevated PSA level and a subsequent biopsy). He knew about all the options and made a preliminary decision to go with active surveillance.

Uh, not so fast. Here is Paul's story.

"Active surveillance is not an option," he was told in no uncertain terms by his fiancée, Andra.

"She's a little more fact based than I am," says Paul. "I tend to be a little . . . airy. She did the research and determined that radiation would be best. So that's what I did."

Andra believed that radiation would do a better job than surgery of sparing the nerves involved with sexual activity. That might not be statistically proven, but Paul's age made him a good candidate for radiation. Indeed, both his potency and his continence returned to almost normal.

"Everything held up for about four years, which was perfect for newlyweds, until my PSA readings started going up. One time the reading went all the way up to 53. Then it came back down to 20. Then it went up again. Crazy. All over the place. Yet whenever I would have a CT scan there would be no sign of any more cancer. Nobody seems to have any idea why my PSAs are so scattered."

Because of the scary readings, Paul was given a prescription for leuprorelin (Lupron), which temporarily shuts down testosterone production. Shut down the testosterone and you shut down the growth of cancer cells, just as castration did when it was used to halt metastatic prostate cancer decades ago. Paul also takes ketoconazole, a synthetic antifungal medication that also has been found to suppress testosterone production.

But Lupron is the one that has really changed his life because it comes with its own carnival of potential side effects—just about anything you can think of, including painful or difficult urination, loss of bowel or bladder control, testicular pain, impotence, and loss of libido. Paul has avoided most of those except for the last one, the one that he had felt so good about maintaining after the initial radiation.

"I still feel I'm in a pretty good place," says Paul. "I work five days a week, still go to the gym. The medication leaves me a little tired, but I'm okay.

"However, there is no way you get an erection with Lupron. You ask me to choose between ice cream and sex these days, and I'm going with ice cream. Trust me, it wasn't that way before."

TAKEAWAY: Lupron can produce "PSA bounce" or "PSA flare." Numbers can also fluctuate because of BPH or prostatitis (inflammation of the gland). But with PSA readings that skyrocket to the levels Paul's have, there is also a possibility that the cancer was not eradicated by the initial radiation. "The most accurate way of determining whether or not cancer remains in the prostate is a biopsy," says Dr. C., the Penn radiation oncologist.

There are many possible causes for wildly varying PSA readings. And let me repeat the mantra of this book: I am not a doctor. Paul's doctors know more than I do. I hope it gets worked out.

Mike Ordille

AGE AT DIAGNOSIS: 62; no cancer

PSA LEVEL: Rose to 2.7, then fell back to 1.7

GLEASON SCORE AND BIOPSY REPORT: First biopsy inconclusive, second biopsy negative

DECISION: No intervention

OUTCOME: So far, so good

I included Mike's experience even though he was not ultimately diagnosed with prostate cancer. Many other men have shared his confounding experience. Here is Mike's story.

"I got yearly checkups and my PSA was always in the 1.7 range, but in 2010 it shot up to 2.7. I had always heard that was okay, but my family doctor strongly recommended that I see a urologist because of the elevation. The urologist advised me that, even though my PSA was low, there was still a chance that I had prostate cancer. So, I could either wait and see or have a biopsy.

"But the mere mention of 'prostate cancer' planted the seed in my brain, and I started thinking, 'My God. I have prostate cancer.'

"The biopsy, which I had in August of 2010, was very painful and something that I wouldn't want to go through again. But though it came out negative for prostate cancer, the urologist said that there were areas of my prostate that were 'suspicious.'

"'*Suspicious*'? What the heck does that mean? They told me that they could keep on monitoring the situation or give me another biopsy. Of course I didn't want another biopsy, but remember that seed that was planted: I might have prostate cancer.

"So I agreed to another biopsy in September. Biopsy day arrived and I wasn't feeling all that great, fever and chills, and, worst of all, burning during urination. What was going on? My wife wanted me to reschedule, but the doctor said, 'Oh, he'll be fine.' I agreed to it because of that I-want-to-know-now mentality.

"The procedure wasn't nearly as bad as the first biopsy, not even close. It was almost like they knew how bad the first one was and decided 'There's probably no cancer there, so let's not be too rough with him and just take the money and run.' Once again I got the news that no prostate cancer was detected, and, obviously, I thought it was behind me.

"But in November the burning with urination started again and didn't stop. I ended up in the emergency room with a high fever, vomiting, and diarrhea. It took a long, long while to make a diagnosis, but finally they found that I had contracted *E. coli* from the first biopsy. So when I went for the second biopsy, rather than find out what was wrong with me, they exposed me to more infection. The infectious disease doctor put me on a strong antibiotic and soon afterward I was released.

"I eventually ended up seeing a urologist at Thomas Jefferson University Hospital in Philadelphia, and he couldn't understand why my treatment was so aggressive. I haven't had another biopsy, my PSA has stayed around 1.7, and things are just fine."

TAKEAWAY: Mike's story illustrates the ultimate biopsy nightmare: Undergo a procedure that is painful, fails to uncover cancer, and—worst of all—unleashes harmful bacteria in your body.

And then be asked to repeat the procedure the following month.

Men are given antibiotics prior to a prostate biopsy. Pre-biopsy, I was given ceftriaxone, and the biopsy needles themselves are treated with an antibiotic. But as Dr. Walsh says, "Today, many patients have antibiotic resistance to drugs like Cipro because of their widespread use, and some patients develop a serious infection despite antibiotic treatment." Dr. Lee, while hopeful about the antibiotic-coated biopsy needle research going on in Israel, describes the situation thusly: "Very scary."

Reasonable minds can disagree—and do—on the wisdom of getting a biopsy based on a PSA of 2.7. But it seems obvious that Mike did not need it. The elevated reading could've come from a lot of things that were not cancer. His PSA has come back down to 1.7 and stayed there.

George Yasso

AGE AT DIAGNOSIS: 50

PSA LEVEL: 800

GLEASON SCORE AND BIOPSY REPORT: None; disease ruled terminal at detection

DECISION: Chemotherapy, radiation, and dietary and alternative treatments

OUTCOME: Fatal

Two decades ago, George and I coached youth basketball for different teams from the same club in Bethlehem, Pennsylvania. George was also president of the club and proved to be that rare person who cared about everybody. His own son, Hank, was a terrific athlete, but on many occasions George gave the practice time that could've gone to Hank's team to other teams. Trust me: That almost never happens in the my-kid-is-all-that-matters world of youth sports.

One of George's younger brothers, Bart, is a well-known running ambassador for *Runner's World* magazine. Bart battled alcohol and drug use as a teenager, and it was his big brother who turned him around. "George gave me the tools," says Bart. "He put me on the right path. He was like a father to me."

This sounds like something you say about someone when he's gone, but it happens to be true: George Yasso made everybody around him better.

Here is George's story.

"George didn't have any fear of doctors or anything like that, but he only went when he needed to," says George's brother Gerry, one of seven kids born to Rose Marie and George F. Yasso, a foreman at Bethlehem Steel. "He always played hurt [George was a football star at Hofstra University and played rugby until his late 30s], and that's how he lived his life. But he took care of himself. He watched his diet and he worked out five days a week. It wasn't like he let himself go."

In the spring of 2001, George was feeling so bad and had lost so much weight that he went to the doctor. "Upper respiratory infection" was one diagnosis. He continued to slide, and finally his wife, Jean, practically dragged him back to the doctor. For the first time in his life he got a digital rectal exam and a PSA test. His level was 800. His cancer had metastasized and was already at stage IV.

"Even then, if you asked George how he felt his answer was always the same," says Jean. " 'Fine,' he would say, 'I feel fine.' "

George kept the news quiet, not telling even his parents or his son and two daughters. "It was the way George did everything," says Jean. "He picked his team, made his plan, and that was it."

George's battle to keep his diagnosis of terminal prostate cancer from becoming public knowledge wasn't successful, however. He was an extremely popular and well-known guy around Bethlehem and word got out, though not always in the right way. Another brother, James (better known as Spud), learned that George had cancer when, in an egregious violation of George's right to privacy, a doctor told him during a checkup. One of George's daughters found out when a blabby technician came out after reading George's scan and announced, "Oh, he has cancer." And his treatment wasn't without mishap, either: During one chemo treatment, an inattentive nurse inserted the IV incorrectly and George got severe burns all the way up his arm.

By the time I found out that George was sick, he had been through chemo and radiation and was deep into alternative treatments. I remember his describing to me a particularly involved series of enemas he was getting. He didn't tell me in so many words that he thought he could beat prostate cancer, but I knew that's what he believed.

"It was in George's head from the moment he was born," says Gerry, "that he could beat anything."

From time to time his PSA went down because of the medication, once all the way to 3, but then it went back above 300. It was a constant series of ups and downs, but through it all George kept his good spirits. One July morning he reported for chemo wearing his golf cleats, got his treatment, and went directly to walk a round of golf.

"He told me to help him up a hill on the last hole," remembers Gerry, "and when we got to the top he said, 'Okay, let go of my arm.' He didn't want anyone to see him getting help."

The course of George's disease was inexorable and hard to watch. This once vital man who could talk the shell off a hard-boiled egg was sometimes rendered speechless by growing tumors. This line-busting fullback kept falling down because of tumors that threw off his balance. When it was obvious he was near the end, George still refused hospice treatment and refused to make a will. "If I do that," George told his family, "I'll be giving up." A lawyer came to his bedside and he did it the day before he died—November 13, 2003.

After such ordeals, family members cling to little blessings. George had gotten one cancer-free year to watch his son Hank play linebacker for the University of New Hampshire. "At 6:00 p.m. on the night he died," remembers Jean, "George was lying in bed watching game films with Hank. He could barely speak, but he was trying to make some point or another about defense. He died three hours later."

With thousands of others, I stood in line for hours at the viewing. Five busloads of coaches, teammates, and parents came from New Hampshire. The Yasso family received visitors for 11 hours.

I ask Jean to look back and come up with one word to describe how she feels.

"Cheated," she says after thinking for a moment. "And not just me. My kids got cheated. Their children will get cheated because they'll never know a man who would've been the greatest grandfather ever. The community got cheated for the things that George will never be able to do. And I got cheated because I'm missing the best person I ever knew."

"One thing George told me before he died has stuck with me," says Gerry. "He said, 'There's a lot of things I still wanted to do, and I regret that I won't get them done. But one regret I don't have? I spent enough time with my kids. I feel very connected to them.'"

That's as fine a final thought as any I've ever heard.

TAKEAWAY: As with Jack Littley and so many others, both sides of the PSA debate could claim George Bartholomew Yasso as Exhibit A.

The USPSTF and its supporters would say that George's cancer was so virulent from the outset that no screening test would've saved him.

Those in favor of PSA testing would say that if George had been screened when he was 40 or even 45, perhaps his PSA would've been elevated and he might've gotten treatment that would've saved his life.

Jean Yasso knows what side she's on.

"I don't want my son waiting until he's 50 to be tested," she says. "It was very frustrating back then because nobody talked about prostate cancer. It wasn't like breast cancer, where there were fund-raisers and awareness months. There was a time—and I remember this—when a woman went to her doctor and whatever he said was what she did. 'Oh, it's nothing, just a little lump.' Well, that changed. It has to change for prostate cancer, too."

CHAPTER 16

...In which the author ponders the lessons of prostate cancer, offers tentative advice, and breaks bread with his prostatectomy pal

THE DAYS TURNED INTO WEEKS, the weeks turned into months, and this sentence turned into something out of a cheesy romance novel. But you get the point. Time marched on as it always does. From March through November 2012 I buried myself in prostate cancer research and interviews to the point where I almost forgot that I had had the disease myself.

All right, that's a bit of a leap. Six days out of 7, maybe 13 out of 14, it's easy to forget. Yes, intimate encounters are different, mainly because they now involve ED medication and are therefore arranged with the precision of Prussian parades. Spontaneity is a possibility, but not the watchword.

But I have no symptoms of disease. I have had two PSA reading since my surgery and both were near zero. My urinary function is normal. Pads are a distant memory. I can't even get mileage out of my abdominal scars, which are all but invisible, save for the small one above my navel through which my bagged and walnut-sized prostate was removed.

I have learned some things—a lot of things—about prostate cancer, which only made me realize how much I don't know. All of those little snapshots that a man with prostate cancer must collect—the results of digital rectal exams, PSA tests, a biopsy, Gleason scoring, an MRI, a bone scan—are exactly that: snapshots. Only when viewed together do they form an intricate mosaic that requires interpretation by a medical professional.

But I sure as hell have formed some opinions, about both my own treatment and the prostate cancer world in general. I offer them here for men who have been diagnosed and don't know what direction to turn in and men who have already had intervention that resulted in positive, negative, or in-between results.

Diet, nutrition, fitness, and lifestyle play a major part in the prostate cancer picture.

Rare is the cancer book—indeed, any health-related book—that these days fails to address the importance of general health in combating and recovering from illness. That doesn't mean it wasn't overdue. "I went through four years of medical school, six years of urology training, and had an oncology fellowship," says Dr. Aaron Katz, "and during that whole time I heard maybe 30 minutes on the role of diet." But it is an emerging field of study. For more information, I direct you to, among other publications, Dr. Katz's *Definitive Guide to Prostate Cancer*. In it, he discusses what he considers to be health-enhancing and cancer-fighting foods for the prostate and even includes a section on how to eat a pomegranate. Another book, this one by Mark Moyad, MD, is called *Promoting Wellness for Prostate Cancer Patients*. Even Dr. Patrick Walsh, who was trained traditionally, details extensive diet and lifestyle information in his *Guide to Surviving Prostate Cancer*.

If you feel good going into a prostate procedure, you have a better chance of feeling good coming out of it. I firmly believe that's part of the reason I recovered so quickly (along with the skill of the surgeon, of course). It's simple logic: The quicker you get up after surgery, the quicker you will recover—that's just a fact—and you will not be able to do that if you're out of shape. I think back to my 137 circuits around the downstairs perimeter when I had my catheter in—it helped me not only physically, but also mentally. In bed, I felt imprisoned; up and out, I felt alive. And it goes beyond "feeling." *Cancer Epidemiology, Biomarkers & Prevention,* an online publication, recently published a study showing that being overweight or obese increased the chances of getting prostate cancer by 57 percent.

But beating cancer, as I (presumably) have, should not be mistaken as a test of character. In a perceptive January 21, 2013, post about disgraced cyclist Lance Armstrong on Salon.com, Samuel G. Freedman, a Columbia University journalism professor and member of the Prostate Cancer Club, wrote the following: "His [Armstrong's] success fit into a certain pervasive narrative of cancer—that cancer is something you 'defeat,' something you 'beat,' less a disease than a test of character. We didn't want to ask exactly how Lance Armstrong, recovering from testicular cancer, could possibly become the top cyclist in the entire world, because the image of his resurrection was, in a nearly religious way, irresistible."

Doctors have agendas, just like everyone else in the world does.

Let me reiterate that I couldn't be more pleased with the medical care I received all the way through this process. But since doctors and surgeons routinely perform such seemingly incredible feats, there is the temptation to look at them as a kind of stethoscope-wielding Justice League of America, superintelligent, superpowered, superknowledgeable. But the vast majority of them are tethered to medical institutions, free-floating entities with decision-making power, to be sure, but not completely divorced from either self-interest or the interests of those who employ them.

"There are all sorts of incentives in the health care system, and I think it's important for patients to understand that," says Dr. John Christodouleas. "At Penn, for example, we are motivated to suggest active surveillance only because it might be good practice."

Translation: As far as the bean counters are concerned, active surveillance, which is not a money-making proposition, is about as attractive as bloodletting with leeches. Active surveillance doesn't pay for da Vinci robots and proton beam machinery.

"In no way, shape, or form is the field of urology incentivized for patients to get radiation," Dr. C. said. "Urologists will benefit more by [patients] getting surgery, in the same way I benefit more when a patient gets radiation. We are partners [he means urologists and radiation oncologists], and to an extent, that keeps us honest. If somebody is flagrantly violating standards, it would be noticed and would affect their professional standing.

"But, look, there are perverse medical incentives everywhere, in every country. You cannot set up a system in which everybody is perfectly aligned with the incentives of the patient. As long as the patient knows where it's perverse, and as long as the physicians try to control themselves, be transparent, and give good reasons for the choices they are making, you will be okay."

To reiterate, I feel that that's what happened with me all along the road. But do not surrender your right to choose. Listen to the experts and weigh not only what they are saying but also why they are saying it, and you should be able to make a reasoned decision.

And so . . .

Get more than one opinion and solicit the advice of survivors.

The wisdom of that is axiomatic for any medical procedure, but even more important with regard to prostate cancer because of the volume of disagreement in the field. True, the farrago of options thrown at you—one doc advocates surgery, another pushes radiation, a third counsels active surveillance—will leave you feeling like you're staring at Bloomberg TV, with all of its competing little boxes. But you have to do it. You have to hear the whole story and you will only get it from different doctors. My interview subjects who had bad outcomes all regret having listened to only one voice.

Also, ask your doctor to give you the names of some of his patients to contact. He has to first check with them, obviously, but he should have nothing to hide. And I've found that, contrary to popular belief, men will talk about prostate cancer and surrender their deepest secrets of the bedroom and bathroom.

You can go to the Internet, of course, and hear scores of endorsements for this modality or that modality. But beware of them because, first of all, there is a lot of misinformation out there, and second, the true believers might be getting paid for their praise.

Keep on reading, but don't believe everything you read, and understand that we are all creatures of our time.

The prostate cancer field is changing constantly. The American Urological Association, which was initially vehemently opposed to the USPSTF recommendation against PSA screening, has now recommended that men under 55 years and at "average risk" to get prostate cancer (i.e., no hereditary connection, not African-American) not be screened. According to a *New York Times* story, more than a dozen companies have either introduced, or are planning to introduce, tests that are more sophisticated and might supplement the PSA test. "Some of the tests are aimed at reducing the false alarms, and accompanying anxiety, caused by elevated PSA readings," the *Times* reported. "Others, intended for use after a definitive diagnosis, examine the genetic workings of the cancer to distinguish dangerous tumors that need treatment from slow-growing ones that might be left alone."

Researchers are working on better biopsies, clearer imaging, ways to make connections to heredity, predictions based on DNA, and a hundred other things. I read about a Harvard study that found that drinking six or more cups of coffee per day reduces the risk of getting any kind of prostate cancer by 20 percent and the risk of developing aggressive forms by 60 percent. (Never mind what it might do for constipation.) There is a highly competitive and emulous scramble to find the Next Big Thing in prostate cancer, and that is invariably accompanied by a tendency to overcelebrate breakthroughs and vastly exaggerate triumphs.

For example, on the Web site for a chain of proton beam treatment centers called ProCure, a headline reads "Proton Therapy May Reduce Risk of Erectile Dysfunction" and a subhead further proclaims: "Prostate Cancer: 94% of men remained sexually active after treatment with proton therapy."

First of all, yes, it may reduce erectile dysfunction. And I may be asked to stand in for Brad Pitt tomorrow. (All right, bad example.) Also, "sexually active" doesn't necessarily mean you have an erection; as thousands of men without prostates know, you can have an orgasm without an erection. And "sexually active" could mean you're indulging in self-inflicted orgasm. In the fine print the report also says that these were men ages 55 and under, which, across the prostate cancer population, is not only a relatively young age to have intervention, but also a young age to undergo radiation.

If something meaningful happens in prostate cancer, something that could truly affect your choice of whether to wait or have intervention, rest assured that those Web sites devoted to prostate cancer will have that news. So will, among others, the Web sites of the *New England Journal of Medicine,* Johns Hopkins University, the Cleveland Clinic, the University of Pennsylvania, and several others listed in Sources and Resources in the back of this book. Make sure you choose reputable sites for information gathering.

At some point, you may have to pull the trigger on a decision, and you can't beat yourself up over what might come along later. In 40 years of covering athletes, the unhappiest ones I encountered were those who constantly inveighed against being born too early and raged that the younger generations made more money than they did. I always wanted to tell those guys, *Look, had you been born earlier, you would've been chasing around mastodons for your winter wardrobe, so put a sock in it.*

When you get your Gleason score, realize that your cancer might be slightly worse.

The prostate biopsy is, to some extent, a shot in the dark—6 to 12 shots in the dark, really. It does not provide a complete picture. "Needles sample 1/1,000th of the prostate," says Dr. Walsh. "There's a vast amount that hasn't been sampled, and oftentimes that cancer is right down where the urethra is, at what's called the apex, the hardest place to get a needle on."

Dr. Walsh estimates that 25 percent of men have more cancer than is shown by the biopsy. That happened to me—my 3 + 3 Gleason was scored at 3 + 4 after the prostate was taken out. Several men I talked to reported the same thing.

No, that doesn't mean I was close to dying. Rare is the cancer scored a 6 that turns out to be a 9 or 10. But it still means that the cancer was a little more serious, and Dr. Walsh believes that the next big step for prostate cancer must come in the field of imaging.

"If we can get to the point where we say, 'Okay, you have Gleason 6 in only a tiny place in your prostate,'" says Dr. Walsh, "yes, we can have a way to diagnose that and monitor it. But we don't have that type of imaging right now."

Whatever your opinions are about intervention, go to the tables.

Let's say you're 65 years old, your PSA is below 4, your Gleason score is 3 + 3, and your biopsy shows localized cancer that has not escaped the prostate. You want to do active surveillance but need that last little bit of convincing. Go to the prediction tables. One of the interviewees in the previous chapter (Bob Snyder) spoke about the one on the Sloan-Kettering Web site, and there's one from Johns Hopkins, too; both are listed in Sources and Resources.

It is easy to use. I put in my PSA (3.8), my Gleason (6), and my clinical stage (T1c), hit FIND RESULTS, and instantly was told the following: My chance of having organ-confined disease was 87 percent. My chance of having cancer that had spread outside my prostate was 12 percent. And my chance of having either seminal vesicle or lymph node involvement was zero.

All in all, that's a bet anyone would make in Vegas—but one I chose not to make with my body. Given the same set of circumstances, you might choose differently.

If you choose intervention, experience counts.

I had excellent success with robotic surgery. But if for some reason I had been given the choice of robotic with an inexperienced surgeon or any other treatment modality (radiation, radioactive seeds, cryotherapy) with a veteran, I would have taken the latter in a heartbeat. The more repetitions of a procedure a surgeon or radiologist does, the more times he or she encounters something that might be a problem, and the more efficient he or she is at dealing with it.

Communicate with your partner and figure out a way to make sex a positive.

This is for those of you who have had intervention and are now experiencing erectile dysfunction. You know who you are. Your partner knows who you are. Your urologist knows who you are because he or she has asked you about it. It's a medical reality, not a congenital weakness or a failure of the will.

You have to talk about it at home. If you stop talking about ED, then it starts to grow and grow (unlike your penis) and becomes this crushing invisible weight that nobody wants to deal with, and the next thing you know, sex has become a hazy memory, like the antics of a particularly adorable pet you used to have.

There are all kinds of statistics out there, but after all my research and interviews I believe what Dr. Pablo Torre says about it. "If people say they get 90 percent of their erection function back, they are probably lying," he says. "Even in the best of hands, ED response is probably about 60 percent to 65 percent. It's much more an issue than continence, which is probably close to 90 percent."

As of this writing, 13 months after surgery, I can get a full erection. Maintaining it is sometimes the problem, a condition known as "venous leak." (Cruelly, "venous" is pronounced like "Venus," the goddess of love, and rhymes with "penis.") In a venous leak, the veins in the penis, diminished by age and weakened by surgery, cannot prevent blood from exiting, stage left, during an erection. Anxiety can also bring it on. You start thinking about a possible failure and next thing you know, it's a self-fulfilling prophecy, what the medical profession calls an example of "psychogenic erectile dysfunction." In the immortal words of Yogi Berra, "Ninety percent of this game is half mental."

But I am working on it and I am optimistic. And there are small benefits. Sometimes the orgasm doesn't feel complete, so I feel like engaging in Act II—something that hadn't happened for many years. And apparently there are other avenues to explore. To combat venous leak, Dr. Walsh (who turns out to be the urological equivalent of Masters and Johnson, by the way) suggests attempting sexual activity standing up. "The escaping blood has to travel all the way back up to the heart, and this takes longer if a man is standing up than if he's lying down," writes Dr. Walsh. Stand-up sex presents interesting possibilities, but also the possibility of a spectacular orthopedic catastrophe.

My wife and I have turned our encounters (none of which, to this point, have occurred vertically) into mini-ceremonies. There is a time for them and a certain ritual they follow, and even if they some-times do not produce volatility, they produce much intimacy, and I do not want to make them a thing of the past. As Jackson Browne wrote in "Running on Empty," "Gotta do what you can just to keep your love alive."

There are surgical remedies for ED, as well as the pumps described in previous chapters. I have nothing against pumps in principle, and I can't be sure that I wouldn't have used one if I were 10 years younger. But I can safely say that a pump is not in my future plans, even if my potency never returns to presurgical levels. It just doesn't fit my men-tal picture of sex, conjuring up as it does images of clogged sinks and water-filled basements. And a needle through my penis to increase blood flow? That just isn't going to happen, either.

If you are so inclined, join a support group and talk about it.

I have attended the meetings of two prostate groups and, to be honest, I went only for research. Journalists tend to be nosy rather than soul-searchingly communicative, and I have not returned.

But if I were suffering from serious postsurgical complications or depression, I would go back in a minute. At both meetings there was a free exchange of ideas, and the participants seemed to get a lot out of them. At one of the meetings I learned that several of the men had been attending for more than a decade. They had become prostate pals, and in their anecdotal exchanges one feeling came to the fore:

I am not alone.

That is very important.

Anyway, I don't have much left to talk about. I've been talking for the last 190 pages. That's a lot of catharsis for one man.

I would make the same treatment decision again. I'm almost sure I would. My decision-making process was absolutely impeccable. Unless it wasn't. But I'm sure . . .

I have tried to make sense of the studies and statistics used by both sides in the PSA debate, and I have dutifully called and e-mailed both sides many times for clarifications. My in-box is bulging with the replies of Dr. Walsh, Dr. T. Ming Chu, Dr. David Lee, Dr. Keith Van Arsdalen, Dr. William Catalona, and the USPSTF's Dr. Michael LeFevre. But as I wrote in the Prologue, it boils down to a statistical version of *Rashomon*. The experts look at the same data and extrapolate from them entirely different conclusions, and that's disheartening. I sincerely doubt that the average man would be able to read through the studies and say with certainty: "Okay, I get it."

But here's what I do get:

Overscreening exists. Overdiagnosis exists. Overtreatment exists. As I was finishing this book, the authors of a study published in the *New England Journal of Medicine* reported that routine mammograms have resulted in tumors being detected that would never have led to clinical symptoms in 1.3 million women over the last 30 years.

But I can only tell you that despite the relatively low chance that I would've died from prostate cancer, I would again choose to do what I chose to do in 2011, the Year of Indecision. I would take my "little Gleason 6" and present myself in Operating Room 9 at Penn Presbyterian, where, with David Lee at the robot's controls, I would surrender my 39-gram prostate to the Mayo stand.

Which also means: I am glad I got my PSA taken and glad I had a biopsy that revealed my "little Gleason 6."

In the absence of statistical certainty, one must depend upon feelings, seasoned as they might be with a teaspoon of ambivalence. Is my

conclusion influenced by my having had a skilled surgeon, a good outcome, and an understanding wife? Of course. If urine were running
down my leg and I was facing a life bereft of sexual activity, would my
feelings be different? Absolutely.

But after all my interviews and research, three salient facts stay
with me:

1. **THE PEOPLE I MET WHO ARE INVOLVED IN PROSTATE
    CANCER TREATMENT ARE SINCERE AND DEDICATED.**
    Some of them have devoted their professional lives to
    researching and treating this baffling disease. They might
    have, as the saying goes, "skin in the game," but I do not
    believe that, as a group, cashing in on PSA tests and
    needless interventions is what moves those intimately
    involved with other men's prostates. You don't spend
    your life studying this half-buried gland, one that Dr.
    Walsh declares does "much more harm than good," just
    to hear the ring of a cash register.

    That doesn't mean I dismiss the USPSTF entirely. But
    numbers are open to interpretation and interpretations
    are open to interpretation, and at the end of the day your
    thoughts about PSA will probably come down to a matter
    of degree. If you edge over to the traditional corner, where
    Dr. Catalona stands in a white lab coat, you believe that it
    just might save your life. If you edge over to the USPSTF
    corner, where Dr. LeFevre stands holding a calculator, you
    will focus on its inaccuracy and possible deleterious
    effects. But keep in mind that even a doctor like Aaron
    Katz, who chastises Dr. Catalona for relying too heavily
    on the PSA test, routinely uses it himself in diagnosing
    patients. The idea of throwing it out entirely, which is
    what the panel recommends, strikes me as moronic.

2. **THERE ARE MEN SUFFERING FROM PROSTATE CANCER WHO DO NOT DIE OF IT.** The USPSTF presents the debate as if it were a zero-sum game, i.e., you live or you die, and, according to the panel, only slightly more of those who are not PSA tested die than those who are PSA tested.

    But there are men with advanced metastatic prostate cancer who might not die from it. They might be 90 and die of a heart attack, but when they were alive they still had prostate cancer. And despite the inkling of doubt I have, no one could ever convince me that there was no chance I wouldn't have developed advanced prostate cancer when I was, say, 75. I didn't want that to happen. Too many other things will happen to me, so I'd rather have one less thing to worry about.

3. **HUMAN BEINGS HAVE A REMARKABLE ABILITY TO ADAPT TO OUTCOMES THAT ONCE WOULD'VE SEEMED TRAGIC.** Poorly executed or inappropriate interventions and cursed bad luck have most assuredly led men down the road of impotence and incontinence, but, statistically, how often does that happen? I don't think that often across the population. And for the men in that vast fraternity (Phi Prosta Gonna) who have some incontinence and some erectile dysfunction, how many would say that those outcomes are acceptable to have rid themselves of cancer? I would say a lot.

    "With regard to prostate cancer, no man can predict what incontinence or impotence might mean for him," wrote Pamela Hartzband, MD, and Jerome Groopman, MD, in an excellent opinion piece published in the September 13, 2012, issue of the *New England Journal of Medicine* and headlined "There Is More to Life Than Death." "There is often a profound disconnect between the way healthy people view medical conditions and the way patients with these conditions view themselves."

Ten years from now there might be a new way of looking at PSA. Perhaps researchers will have found conclusive evidence that a man tested at 50 whose PSA reading is below, say, 1, will have almost zero chance of getting metastatic prostate cancer and therefore won't have to be tested again, or biopsied, irradiated, or cut open. The research and endless debate will continue, and I will continue to listen and hope that I don't have buyer's regret. But as I write this, here's one thing I don't have: prostate cancer.

ON A BRISK NOVEMBER DAY I meet Leonard Collier at a Center City Philadelphia restaurant. We have the instant kinship of sailors who had been on a rocky voyage but returned to shore safely.

"The last time I saw you, Leonard," I say, "you were naked with your legs spread. You look a helluva lot better now."

We are at a steakhouse, but he orders grilled fish and I get lobster salad. We have both pledged to stay on top of our physical conditioning.

"I had about five months to prepare for the operation," says Leonard. "I took long walks, got my core in shape. I think it made a difference. And I followed the postsurgery instructions to the letter."

He pulls out two pieces of paper bearing post-op instructions. Each numbered item—"If constipated, drink lots of fluids, expect incontinence and impotency for several months," for example—has been highlighted with a yellow marker, and some have annotations.

"I was an educator, Jack, and I'm always organized," says Leonard.

One of those annotations says "Yippee!" next to it. It was the date of his first successful sexual encounter with Asha.

"There it is," he says. "Surgery, October 3; October 24, full erection for orgasm. I had taken Cialis on Monday the 22nd. This was two days later."

"You really defied the odds on that one, Leonard," I tell him.

"As soon as it was over, Asha says, 'We have to call Jack.' So she did."

"I am truly honored you made me your first call, Leonard," I tell him.

I ask Leonard to sketch out his prostate specifics. He had it all down. His PSA, which he had always gotten tested for his yearly physicals, had in three years crept from 3.99 to 4.2 to 5.2. The biopsy showed two involved cores with a Gleason of 3 + 3 on one and 3 + 4 on the other. That was enough for him.

"Again, I did my homework," says Leonard. "I knew that African Americans are at a higher risk for prostate cancer than white men. My grandfather had prostate cancer—I don't know if he died from it—and my father [William Collier] has it right now. He's 87. He's had radiation treatments. It's been up and down for him.

"And I talked to friends. Out of 20 of my golfing buddies, 8 had either an enlarged prostate or had had surgery. There was plenty of prostate conversation. And it was good because a lot of time black men don't like to talk about what's going on down there, about sexual life and leakage and things like that."

"A lot of times white men don't either, Leonard," I say. "But I found in my research that a lot do, too. It surprised me." He also talked to his daughter, Monique, a pediatrician, and she advised him to take action. "So I decided that surgery was the way to go," says Leonard. "I did my homework and made three appointments with surgeons. Dr. Lee was first. After I talked to him I canceled the other two. That's how strongly I felt about him."

I ask Leonard if he has heard the drumbeat about active surveillance and the USPSTF recommendation against PSA testing.

"Yes, I read all about it and heard all about it, and it didn't affect me one bit," he says. "My Gleason was high enough to get it, I was a black man at risk, and that's all there was to it. That doesn't mean I wasn't a little nervous. Do you know I had never been in a hospital before?"

"Man, I have you there," I say. "I've managed to screw up various parts of my body over the years. And I found that, while modern medicine has a hard time keeping schedules straight and keeps harassing you with bills you've already paid, they generally do a helluva job in operating rooms."

"My faith kept me positive," says Leonard. "I had Asha there. She would be my strength."

"I hear you," I said. "Donna did the same for me."

"I came out a few weeks after the operation and beat all my friends in golf. They said, 'That doctor should've kept you in another month. You kicked our ass and took our money.' Then the second round? I couldn't do a thing."

"Same thing happened to me," I say. "Good first outing, lousy second. But you know what? I blamed it on cancer."

"Me, too," says Leonard. "We can do that from now on."

It's time to leave. We promise to keep in touch, get together with our "nurses." I tell Leonard that I feel good for him, not only because he had a good outcome, but also because he feels so absolutely, blessedly confident about it.

"Journalists tend not to be completely optimistic about anything," I say. "We're not happy unless we have doubt. We thrive best in a world of second-guessing."

"Well, I don't have any," Leonard says. "I just wanted to be rid of it. I have a lot to live for. Asha. A wonderful daughter and son. My grandson. I babysit him one week out of the month. I play golf. I travel. I work two days a week at a supermarket just to stay busy. Life is good, you know? I didn't want this hanging over my head. I consider it the best decision I ever made."

We shake hands and depart in different directions, now bound by a disease and a diagnosis, by the skill of a surgeon and the gentle understanding of two women, citizens of a slightly altered physical universe and—the small doubts of one notwithstanding—happy as hell to be walking in it.

Sources and Resources

The Author's E-Mail Address

jacksprostatebook@gmail.com

Books

The Decision: Your Prostate Biopsy Shows Cancer. Now What?,
by John C. McHugh (N/A: Jennie Cooper Press, 2009).

*The Definitive Guide to Prostate Cancer: Everything You Need to Know
about Conventional and Integrative Therapies,* by Aaron E. Katz
(New York: Rodale, 2011).

Dr. Patrick Walsh's Guide to Surviving Prostate Cancer, 3rd edition,
by Patrick C. Walsh and Janet Farrar Worthington (New York: *Grand
Central Life & Style,* 2012).

*Promoting Wellness for Prostate Cancer Patients: A Guide for Men
and Their Families,* 3rd edition, by Mark A. Moyad (Ann Arbor, MI:
Ann Arbor Editions, 2010).

*The Whole Life Prostate Book: Everything That Every Man—at Every Age—
Needs to Know about Maintaining Optimal Prostate Health,*
by H. Ballentine Carter and Gerald Secor Couzens (New York:
Free Press, 2012).

Other Materials

One of many stories from the *New York Times* about the purported harms
of PSA testing: http://www.nytimes.com/2011/10/09/magazine/
can-cancer-ever-be-ignored.html

A story from the *New York Times* about PSA overtesting in elderly men:
http://www.nytimes.com/2011/04/12/health/12prostate.html

An article from the *New England Journal of Medicine* reporting that 15-year death rates were lower with prostatectomy than with active surveillance: http://www.nejm.org/doi/full/10.1056/NEJMoa1011967

The US Preventive Services Task Force recommendation statement: http://www.uspreventiveservicestaskforce.org/prostatecancerscreening/prostatefinalrs.htm

An opinion piece from the *New England Journal of Medicine* about medical choice: http://www.nejm.org/doi/full/10.1056/NEJMp1207052

An article summarizing the findings of a study on the benefits of PSA testing: http://www.webmd.com/prostate-cancer/news/20120730/study-psa-testing-cuts-worst-prostate-cancers

Two different opinions of PSA testing: http://online.wsj.com/article/SB10000872396390444301704577631431570809256.html

A well-known Swedish study that found PSA screening beneficial while also noting the "substantial" risk of overdiagnosis: http://www.researchgate.net/publication/45089772_Mortality_results_from_the_Göteborg_randomised_population-based_prostate-cancer_screening_trial/file/d912f505c4d8364410.pdf

A prostate cancer expert and oncologist discusses prostate cancer: http://www.scientificamerican.com/article.cfm?id=prostate-cancer-screening-and-treatments

Much-debated op-ed from Richard Ablin, MD, about the PSA test: http://www.nytimes.com/2010/03/10/opinion/10Ablin.html

A rebuttal to Dr. Ablin by James Mohler, MD, of the Roswell Park Cancer Institute: http://www.roswellpark.org/media/news/psa-and-psa-test-what-public-needs-know

More on the Dr. Ablin op-ed from John McHugh, MD, a urologist: http://theprostatedecision.wordpress.com/about/my-letter-to-the-new-york-times-in-regards-to-richard-albin-discoverer-of-psa

An article from *Men's Health* magazine about a man who regrets surrendering his prostate: http://www.menshealth.com/health/coping-prostate-cancer

Michael Lasalandra, a medical journalist, describes his decision to choose active surveillance: http://www.watchwait.com/my_story.php

Jeff Jarvis's blog on prostate cancer: http://buzzmachine.com/2009/08/10/the-small-c-and-me/

The Prostate Cancer Foundation page on erectile dysfunction: http://www.pcf.org/site/c.leJRIROrEpH/b.5836625/k.75D7/Erectile_Dysfunction.htm

Myths about prostate cancer from the Fred Hutchinson Cancer Research Center: http://www.newswise.com/articles/view/592867/

An article from MedPage Today reporting that a study found that proton beam therapy is not superior to regular radiation: http://www.medpagetoday.com/HematologyOncology/ProstateCancer/32213

The abstract of a paper comparing the biopsy costs and rates of cancer diagnosis of self-referring urologists and urologists who used independent labs: http://content.healthaffairs.org/content/31/4/741.abstract

Another critique of self-referring urologists and their facilities by a private-practice radiation oncologist: http://www.dattoli.com/publication/CHOICESvol27-2june2011.pdf

An article about the link between heredity and prostate cancer: http://www.health.harvard.edu/newsweek/Heredity_and_prostate_cancer.htm

A study about penis length following prostatectomy: http://www.ncbi.nlm.nih.gov/pubmed/12629384

An article from *New York* magazine about longevity: http://nymag.com/news/features/parent-health-care-2012-5

A story about combining BPH drugs with PSA readings to detect aggressive cancer: http://www.sciencedaily.com/releases/2012/08/120809090530.htm

A video about penile prosthesis surgery from the well-regarded Cleveland Clinic: http://www.youtube.com/watch?v=7EVVzUI8s2U

Indispensable Web Sites

American Cancer Society: www.cancer.org

The Cleveland Clinic: http://my.clevelandclinic.org/disorders/prostate_
cancer/hic_prostate_cancer_basics.aspx

Johns Hopkins active surveillance program link:
http://urology.jhu.edu/prostate/advice1.php

Johns Hopkins James Buchanan Brady Urological Institute:
http://urology.jhu.edu

Mayo Clinic:
http://www.mayoclinic.com/health/prostate-cancer/DS00043

MedlinePlus prostate cancer information:
http://www.nlm.nih.gov/medlineplus/prostatecancer.html

Memorial Sloan-Kettering Cancer Center:
http://www.mskcc.org/cancer-care/adult/prostate

Milken Institute: http://www.milkeninstitute.org

National Cancer Institute: www.cancer.gov

National Comprehensive Cancer Network: http://www.nccn.org/index.asp

The New England Journal of Medicine: http://www.nejm.org

NewYork-Presbyterian Hospital/Weill Cornell Medical Center:
http://nyp.org/services/oncology/prostate-cancer.html

Prostate Cancer Foundation:
http://www.pcf.org/site/c.leJRIROrEpH/b.5699537/k.BEF4/Home.htm

The Prostate Net: http://prostatenet.com

Roswell Park Cancer Institute: http://www.roswellpark.org/cancer/prostate

University of Pennsylvania Health System (where the author was treated):
http://www.pennmedicine.org

For families of prostate cancer sufferers: http://www.hisprostatecancer.com

General prostate cancer information from a private network of oncologists:
http://www.prostate-cancer.com

General Web site for men's health issues: http://malecare.org

Online Prostate Cancer Tools

Johns Hopkins Medicine Partin Tables:
   http://urology.jhu.edu/prostate/partintables.php

Memorial Sloan-Kettering Cancer Center Prediction Tools:
   http://www.mskcc.org/cancer-care/adult/prostate/prediction-tools

University of Texas Medicine Cancer Therapy and Research Center:
   http://deb.uthscsa.edu/URORiskCalc/Pages/uroriskcalc.jsp

Acknowledgments

This book never would have gotten started had I not received so many e-mails, calls, and letters after my columns appeared in the Allentown, Pennsylvania, *Morning Call* newspaper. So I would like to thank those people first, some of whom are also mentioned in the book.

In alphabetical order (and I hope I haven't missed anyone):

George Anthony, Henry Bartholomew Jr., Ron Bauer, Fred Bergstresser, Robin Blackburne, Jim Boeheim, John Brinson, Joe Brogan, Lou Burdick, Peter Carry, Mike Caruso, Bruce Charon, Frank Claps, Ken Clifford, Larry Christoff, John Craig, Donna Dowlatshahi, Steve Drescher, David Ernhoffer, Bob Fink.

Brenda Gerhard, Dennis Glew, Richard Grammes, Dana Grubb, Jim Haering, Carol Huennenkens, Gary Jerabek, Robert and Sandy Keiber, Joe Lamack, Jack Littley, David Lubar, Bruce Mack, John Makuvek Jr., Scott Marakovits, Emery Marsteller, Richard Mauthe, Jim Mikitka, Jeff Mohler, Ron Montz.

Norman Morris, Bill and Ann Moss, John Moyer, Robert Murphy, Ken Muth, Paul Newton, Chuck Pinyan, DL (Ron) Pizarie, Ralph Puerta, Jay Radio, Charlie Repka, Paul Rosen, Elmer Ruppert, Gale Siess, Suzzie Silfies, Bob Snyder, Kevin Snyder.

The Spang family, Bill Springer, John Stoffa, Glenn Walbert, Dan Weaver, Bob and Flo Wheeler, Gene Wieder, Joel Wingard, Bob Young, Wayne Young.

Thanks to Rodale Inc. and especially to my editor, Mark Weinstein. Thanks also to copy editor Nancy Elgin, fact-checker Sonya Maynard, and project editor Nancy Bailey. And a shout-out to my agent, Scott Waxman.

I would also like to thank Bob Orenstein and Tim Darragh of the *Morning Call*.

ACKNOWLEDGMENTS

Arnold Palmer gave me a memorable 30 minutes in person and Senator Robert Dole gave me a memorable 20 on the telephone. Jeff Jarvis isn't quite as well known as Arnie or Senator Dole, but he was lot funnier than either of them—and anyone else—during our conversation. Thanks to all three of them.

Though the subject matter wasn't all that pleasant, it was nice spending time with two friends, Jean Yasso and Gerry Yasso, the widow and brother, respectively, of George B. Yasso, to whom this book is dedicated.

And it was great meeting two new friends, Asha Jagtiani and Leonard Collier, my prostatectomy pal.

For expediting interviews and providing general information I'd like to thank Annie Deck-Miller of the Roswell Park Cancer Institute, and to Stacy Loeb, MD, I owe a debt of gratitude for the lengthy interview on SiriusXM Satellite Radio.

Kelly Monahan deserves much applause for her care during my operation, her explanations after it, and her oh-so-gentle removal of you know what.

Nonfiction writing almost always involves asking questions, but I've never been involved in a project where I had to ask so many, the result, obviously, of my being somewhat out of my element when I started. For enlightenment, I needed the experts, who are, in alphabetical order:

Dr. Peter Bach, Dr. Jerry Blaivas, Dr. William Catalona, Dr. John Christodouleas, Dr. T. Ming Chu, Dr. Steven Kaplan, Dr. Aaron Katz, Dr. David Lee, Dr. Michael LeFevre, Dr. James Manley, Dr. Edward Messing, Dr. Pablo Torre, Dr. Keith Van Arsdalen, Dr. Patrick Walsh, and Dr. Samuel Waxman.

Dr. Walsh deserves special notice because of the number of times that he, though a busy man, got back to me with more information. And Dr. Lee deserves special, special attention for doing the same, plus sharing a cheesesteak and fries and a couple rounds of golf and . . . let's see . . . oh, yes, keeping me alive in the OR.

Finally, Donna Lee Kisselbach McCallum nursed me back to health, did much of the research and some of the editing for this book, and endured public conversation of our private life, all with grace and good humor. But after 40 years together, that's hardly a surprise.

—*Stone Harbor, New Jersey, January 2013*

Index

About the Author

Jack McCallum is a veteran sportswriter and the author or coauthor of nine books, including the bestselling *Dream Team* (2012), the critically acclaimed *Seven Seconds or Less,* and collaborations with Shaquille O'Neal and Olympic gold medalist speed skater Dan Jansen. As a writer with *Sports Illustrated* for nearly 30 years, he is best known for his pro basketball coverage, and he also edited the weekly Scorecard section. He is currently a special contributor to the magazine. McCallum won the Curt Gowdy Award from the Naismith Memorial Basketball Hall of Fame in 2005 and before that was awarded the national Women's Sports Foundation Media Award. Today, McCallum teaches journalism at Muhlenberg College, his alma mater, and lives in Bethlehem, Pennsylvania, with his wife, Donna.